Sex and Character

Deborah D. Cole
Maureen Gallagher Duran

William Dembski
Academic Editor

Pandas Publications: A Series About Central Questions from Haughton Publishing Company · Dallas, Texas

Book design: Buell Design

Printed in the United States of America

ISBN 0-914513-50-8
Library of Congress Catalog Card Number: 98-072932

On Thursday, March 19, 1998, local TV weather broadcasts across the southeastern United States warned viewers of impending storms. Widespread conditions ripe for powerful thunderstorms and possibly tornadoes were expected to develop overnight. By Friday morning, twelve people in north Georgia had lost their lives, 91 others were injured, two were missing, 70 to 80 homes were destroyed and 300 more were damaged. A Federal state of emergency was declared for a five county area.

Undoubtedly, advance warning and specific precautionary instruction had saved the lives of many individuals and might have saved more. But the key to this nightmare of destruction was the presence of widespread conditions for which information delivery systems and the individual application of safety instructions were clearly no match.

Today in America's youth culture, widespread conditions are ripe for a different kind of "nightmare of destruction." These conditions have to do with the loss of basic qualities of character and decency. Unfortunately, these conditions will not end in the morning.

Since I opened my obstetrics and gynecology practice in Austin, Texas, in 1968, sexually transmitted disease in America has become epidemic. Three million teenagers, about 25 percent of sexually active teens, are newly infected with a sexually transmitted disease every year.

With *Sex and Character*, the authors and producers have made an enormous contribution to the children of America on behalf of all who care about their welfare. The destruction of our young is no narrow, sectarian concern. Whether black or white, Hispanic or Eastern, Republican or Democrat, liberal or conservative, we all want our children to grow up with sound guidance from the adults in their lives, guidance that will allow them to develop integrity and strong character. We want this for our youth because with the inner strength of sound values, they are less likely to engage in risky behaviors while they are young. As a result, they are more likely to enjoy physical and emotional health, first as young adults and later as mature adults.

Prof. Thomas Lickona, professor of education at the State University of New York at Cortland, director of the Center for the 4th and 5th Rs, and a leader in the character development movement in the United States, often cites ten trends in youth character that are cause for deep concern. Among them are:

1. A rise in youth violence.
2. An increase in dishonesty (lying, cheating, and stealing).
3. An increase in peer cruelty.
4. A growing disrespect for parents, teachers, and other legitimate authority figures.
5. A rise in self-destructive behaviors, such as premature sexual activity, substance abuse, and suicide.
6. The tendency to engage in destructive behavior without thinking it wrong.
7. A rise in prejudice and hate crimes.
8. A decline in basic ethical literacy—including ignorance of moral knowledge as basic as the Golden Rule.

These are the unmistakable symptoms of a youth culture that is breaking away from the morality of even our pluralistic culture at the end of the century. In her book *Reviving Ophelia*, Mary Pipher describes the impact of our youth culture on the lives of teenage girls. She says, "Adolescent girls come of age in a culture preoccupied with money, sex, and violence, a culture with enormous problems—poverty, pollution, addiction, and lethal sexually transmitted diseases.

She adds that "The ways that media have dehumanized sex and fostered violence should be the topic of a national debate." Until Americans develop the grit for that debate, however, the authors and producers of this book are right to address the problem at the level of character. In fact, it must be done. Their work shows the way like a bright floodlight to those who would help guide young people through the stormy night.

As adults use this book, they will not only gain up-to-date insight on why good character is indispensable, but also how to teach it. Young people will learn what good character is and that they can make good values a core part of their innermost character. They will learn that by becoming a person of strong character they can have lives more full of meaning, more free of difficulties, with greater hope for the future.

Dr. Thomas Elkins, chief of gynecologic specialties at Johns Hopkins University, said: "In our current sexually transmitted disease epidemic in America, the message of abstinence until marriage (i.e., committed, lifelong monogamy) has never made more sense. Sadly, growing numbers of those raised in a 'safe sex message' era are filling our clinics. It's definitely time to give abstinence-based, character-focused, peer-taught programs a chance."

I know of no better place to begin than with the use of this book with your students, your own children, your friends, your colleagues, your church or synagogue, your circle of influence, your community, and your state. By spreading the message of this book, you will help our entire culture become a better place for us all, especially for our children.

Joe S. McIlhaney, Jr., M.D.
Austin, Texas

TABLE OF CONTENTS

PTER

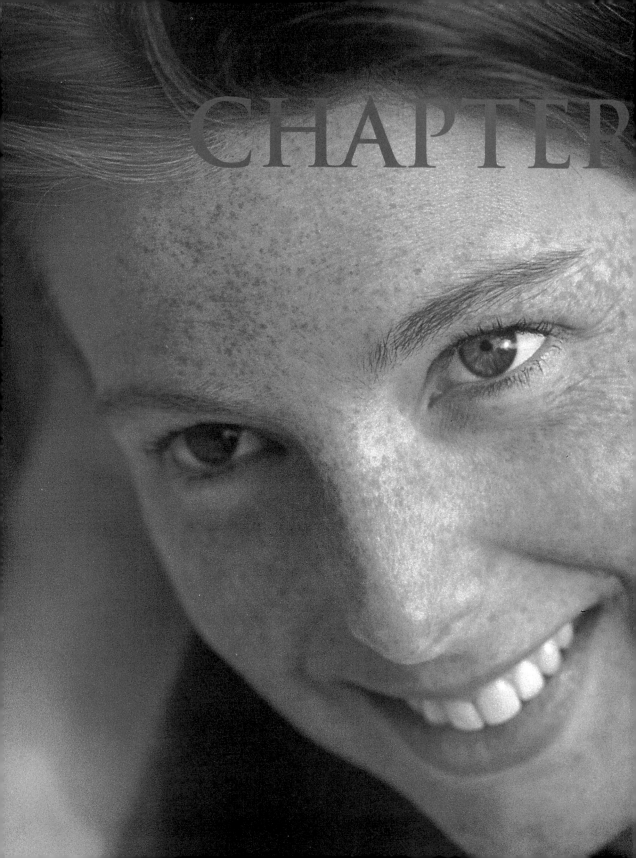

CHAPTER

1

The people's good is the highest law.

SEX, LOVE, AND CHARACTER

-Marcus Cicero, 106–43 B.C.

How far would you go to do what you know is right? Would you sacrifice something important? Would you risk your life? Would you face being ridiculed and rejected?

One person who understood the meaning of sacrifice was Norm Cadarette. In 1983 he contracted HIV (the AIDS virus) from a blood transfusion during open heart surgery. He did not find out until 1987 that he was infected.

Norm knew that no truly safe measures existed to prevent the sexual transmission of HIV and that he could infect his wife, Ginny, with AIDS, as long as they shared sexual intimacy. He loved his wife very much, so he decided to give up having sex with her. Ginny agreed with this decision. She knew that Norm loved her because he was willing to set aside his desire for sex and put her first. After that they remained abstinent.

"True love will never put the object of that love at risk," Norm said.

The Cadarettes gave up physical intimacy, but they still enjoyed a happy, fulfilling marriage. Sex had been only one part of their relationship. They were best friends and shared intimately all the things that were in their hearts.

The Cadarettes learned how true love responds when it confronts a deadly disease. As a family with their daughter,

Jennifer, they refused to focus on themselves and HIV. Instead, Norm and Ginny talked with others about their marriage and how they found intimacy by being best friends. They spoke to as many as 150,000 people a year at schools, colleges, churches, camps, and conferences, helping young people discover what true love means.

"What kids truly want is someone to share their heart with," Ginny said, "and to be a deep part of the other person."

Norm died on April 5, 1995.[1]

Norm Cadarette demonstrated what most people would call *good character*. When his circumstances demanded it, he knew the right thing to do and believed so much in it that he actually did something about it. He gave up the pleasure of sexual intimacy with his wife to protect her from his deadly disease.

Another person who understands the importance of good character is Armstrong Williams. One day his father sent him to town to buy fencing and wire for their farm in South Carolina.

He was sixteen and, under normal conditions, would have jumped at the chance to take the Chevy pickup for a spin. But not this time. His father told him he had to ask for credit.

Armstrong was proud. He wanted respect, not a handout. He'd stood by when his friends asked for credit and waited, with their heads down, while the owner of a store wondered whether they were "good for it." He knew that other young black men were treated like thieves by store clerks every time they entered a grocery store.

The Williams family was honest and paid their debts. But with money scarce just before harvest, Armstrong wondered if the store owner would trust them.

At the general store he carried the items to the register. "I need to put this on credit," he told the man behind the register.

A farmer standing nearby glanced at him skeptically.

The owner replied, "Sure. Your daddy is always good for it." To the farmer he said, "This here is one of James Williams's sons."

The farmer gave an appreciative nod. *James Williams's son.* Those words had paved the way for an adult to respect and trust him.

In that trip to town Armstrong discovered the value of the good name his parents had earned. Because of it the whole family enjoyed their neighbors' respect. The Williamses had a reputation for being decent people who kept their word and respected themselves too much to do something wrong.

Even the ten children—eight boys and two girls—could reap the benefits of that good name without earning it, "unless and until we did something to lose it," Armstrong said. If one child compromised it, the whole family would suffer. "A good name, and the responsibility that came with it, forced us children to be better than we otherwise might be. We wanted to be thought of as good people, and by acting like good people for long enough, we became pretty decent citizens."

Wanting to keep the respect of a good name, Armstrong Williams became the first member of his family to attend college. He later started his own successful public relations firm in our nation's capital.[2]

Someone else who understood good character was high school sophomore Melissa Whitaker. Steve Branson, a senior and the star quarterback on their football team, had asked her for a date. As Saturday night approached, Melissa kept wondering why he had asked her out instead of one of the more popular seniors.

At 7:00 sharp Steve drove up in front of the Whitaker house in his new sports car. Melissa was a little nervous, but Steve's outgoing personality put her at ease. They ate dinner at an expensive restaurant and then drove to a party for football players and their dates. Around midnight, Steve and Melissa said good-bye to the other kids and walked out the door.

"Hey, Mel, why don't I show you where I live?" Steve asked as they reached his car.

"OK," Melissa said quickly. As they entered his house, she wondered if she'd made the right decision. His parents were not at home. But she felt comfortable with Steve. What could go wrong?

The couple sat on the sofa talking and laughing as they watched TV.

After a while Steve leaned over and kissed Melissa.

"Stay with me tonight," he whispered.

Melissa felt her heart race. Thoughts rushed into her mind: "We're not married.... I hardly know him.... What if my parents find out?... What if I stay?... What if I say *no*?" One thought kept coming back: "But this is Steve Branson!" She knew that many of her friends would have jumped at the chance to spend the night with him.

A tiny voice in her heart finally gave Melissa the answer: "No, I couldn't."

The voice was her mother's, saying, as she always had, "I trust you."

That night as she sat on her own bed, Melissa thought about the evening. She felt good. She had followed her conscience. She might have disappointed Steve, but she had not disappointed herself.

Melissa guessed she wouldn't see much of Steve after that, and some of her friends would make fun of her when word got around at school. But she was still glad she had said *no*. It didn't really matter what her friends thought. She knew she had done the right thing.[3]

You may never face the same challenges Norm or Melissa faced, or encounter the racial barriers Armstrong encountered. But you will meet circumstances that test your character—circumstances that show your ability to judge right from wrong and your willingness to act on that knowledge.

The purpose of this book is to help you meet the kinds of challenges these people faced, earn the respect of a good name, and develop good character in your intimate relationships, particularly in the area of sexuality.

Chapter 2 looks at what good character is; why good character is important; and how it is a lifelong pursuit. The chapter includes a section for examining your own

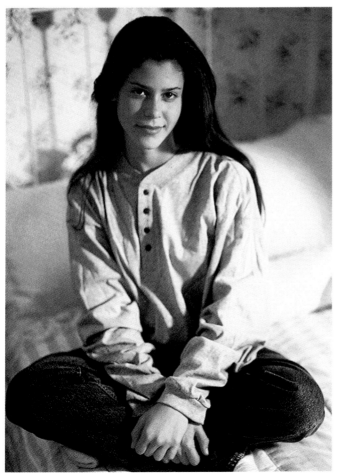

character traits.

Chapter 3 explores character and sexuality, reviewing some of the benefits of good character, as well as highlighting some of the ways people often violate good character in their sexual relationships. Chapters 4, 5, and 6 then look at some of the physical and emotional risks you and your partner run when you have sex before marriage. Chapter 4 discusses sexually transmitted disease. Chapter 5 addresses pregnancy and its consequences. Chapter 6 looks at several emotional consequences of having sex outside of marriage.

Chapter 7 discusses character and dating, showing you how good character can make a difference in your dates and in the quality of your romantic relationships. It also explores some special issues: Is it really love? What if you've already gone too far? This chapter includes two charts: one to help you decide if your relationship is love or infatuation, and another to help you examine your own sexual attitudes and behaviors.

Chapter 8 focuses on character and marriage. It answers questions like: Why does marriage matter? What is the importance of character for marriage?

As Norm Cadarette showed by sacrificing sexual intimacy with his wife, love is more than feelings or self-fulfillment; it is a daily decision. As Armstrong Williams and Melissa Whitaker learned, love means respecting yourself and others so much that you do what is right. Love is about seeking the best for yourself and others—in your words and in your actions. In other words, true love—and that includes the sexual dimension of love—is a matter of character.

1. In the story about Melissa and Steve, Melissa could have avoided the sexual pressure from Steve by making better choices. How could she have avoided the situation with Steve, and what better choices could she have made?

2. Norm Cadarette understood the meaning of love and the value of self-control. He gave up the pleasure of sexual intimacy for the safety and well-being of his wife and daughter. What are the advantages and disadvantages of his decision?

3. What do you think of the following statement: If sexual self-control is impossible prior to marriage, then it will be difficult within marriage.

4. How did you develop a sense of right and wrong? Who and what has influenced your sexual decision-making? How did your mom and dad treat each other? How have your family and childhood experiences influenced your views on human sexuality?

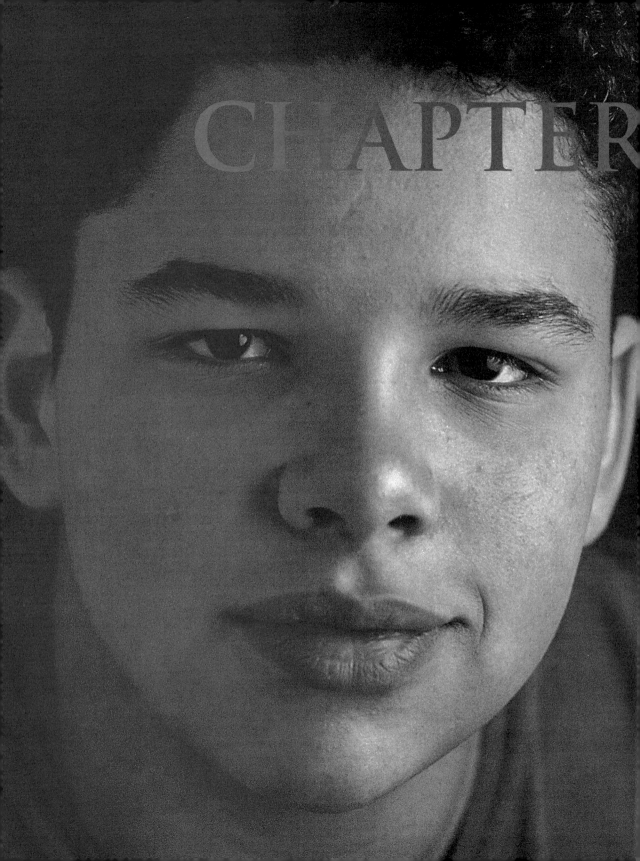

Good Character

-Theodore Roosevelt

Here are four true stories about people who found lost wallets.

In a town in Massachusetts a teenager carrying a skateboard under his arm spotted a wallet on the sidewalk in front of a local pharmacy. He stepped inside the store, purchased a magazine, and handed the wallet to the clerk. "Someone lost this," he said.

On being called, the owner of the wallet hurried to the store and offered the teenager a reward for returning it. But the boy refused to accept it.

"I can't take the money," he said. "I was a schmuck and kept this." He pulled twenty dollars out of his pocket.

This eighteen-year-old had occasional jobs as a landscaper and said the money could have helped pay his rent. "I'm sorry I tried to steal it," he told the wallet's owner. "Morality really messes with you," he said. "But that's a good thing," he added.

A similar incident occurred in Atlanta, Georgia. A woman discovered a wallet in the food court of a busy mall. She almost turned it in to mall security but thought that "maybe somebody would take the money out of it." Instead she called the owner of the wallet. She told him that her parents had taught her to be honest. But she hadn't learned the lesson right away. "I found one

time. I returned it, but I took twenty dollars from it. That twenty dollars bugged me so bad I swore if I ever had the chance again, I'd do the right thing."

The right thing? How do you know what the right thing is? The boy in the first story said he knew because morality "messed" with him. He had an uncomfortable feeling that stealing the money from the wallet was wrong. He acted on that uneasy feeling and returned the money. The woman knew because her parents had taught her about honesty. She had felt bad when she held back twenty dollars from a purse years earlier. Because of that feeling she determined to do the right thing if she ever had a second chance. Both the young man and the woman were learning what it means to have good character.

Here's a third and different story. Dressed in neat blue jeans and a white T-shirt, a young man spied a billfold in front of a Las Vegas hotel. He plucked it off the sidewalk, glancing at the many people passing by. Entering the hotel, he appeared to look around for someone to whom he could hand it. He left that hotel, walked into another, and checked out the security guards there, possibly trying to decide what to do. Outside again, he stuck the wallet in his front pocket and walked on down the street. He passed several policemen and melted into the crowd. The wallet was never returned.

That young man seemed to know it was right to return the wallet to its owner and apparently had feelings about it, but in the end he chose to do what was wrong.

Consider a fourth story. Two teenage boys discovered a wallet in a Los Angeles mall. One boy pulled the money out and whooped. Then they both talked at once as they walked through the mall. After a few minutes they encountered a man who appeared to be one boy's father. They showed him what they had found. The man and the two boys left the mall. The owner of the wallet was never called.

Neither the boys nor the man gave any indication of knowing or caring about what was right.

THE SCORE

These true stories were part of an experiment by the editors of *Reader's Digest*. They wanted to see what Americans would do when faced with a choice of keeping or returning something that did not belong to them. Of 120 wallets "dropped," 80 were returned —about 67 percent. What's more, of the 80 wallets returned, about 55 came back with their contents unchanged.

Of those who returned the wallets,

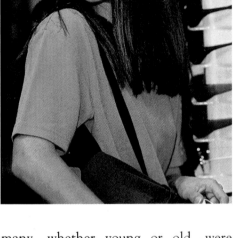

many—whether young or old—were skeptical about the honesty of young people.

"Youngsters are gonna probably keep it," commented one man in Pennsylvania.

"If they're about fourteen to eighteen, they probably wouldn't return it," said a twenty-one-year-old college student in California.

"There are kids who will just take the cash and dump the wallet," asserted an eighteen-year-old in Massachusetts.

As it turned out, ten of the fifteen young people who found the wallets returned them and the money—right in line with the 67 percent average.

Most of the returners in the experiment said that their parents had instilled in them the desire to do the right thing. One thirty-eight-year-old North Carolina man recalled a time when he had shoplifted as a kid. His mother took him back to the store so he could return the candy he had stolen, apologize, and pay for it. "It taught me a big lesson," he said.

The experiment proved that most people still have a conscience—one element of good character—even if they don't always follow it. The ones who meant to keep the money usually glanced about nervously and tried to conceal the wallets. Their actions revealed that they knew they were doing something wrong.[1]

In the first chapter Norm Cadarette, Armstrong Williams, and Melissa Whitaker were three people who demonstrated good character. We saw how sex, love, and character are linked. The purpose of this chapter is to study the components, values, and importance of good character, and to show that character development is a lifelong pursuit. You will also have an opportunity to evaluate your own character traits through a self-examination section at the end of this chapter.

GOOD CHARACTER DEFINED

How would you do if you faced the same circumstances as the people who found the wallets? Would you know the right thing to do? Would you do it?

Do you know what good character is? Developmental psychologist Tom Lickona explains it this way. He calls good character *moral knowing, moral feeling,* and *moral acting.* The woman and the young man in the first two stories demonstrated those three components of good character. They knew what was

right, felt strongly about what was right, and did what was right. In fact, the word *moral* refers to what is right and wrong in a person's behavior. We need all three components of good character—knowing, feeling, and acting—to be morally mature and lead a moral life, even when we face pressure from outside influences or temptation from inside ourselves.

Character is putting one's values into action. The woman who felt bad about taking twenty dollars from a wallet many years earlier put the value of honesty into action when she returned the wallet in the *Reader's Digest* experiment. Over the years that value became a virtue, a reliable inner disposition to respond to situations in a morally good way. In chapter 1, the tiny voice inside Melissa's heart—her conscience—illustrated this reliable inner disposition; it helped her respond to Steve's sexual pressure in the right way.

Let's look more closely at the three essential components of good character: moral knowing, moral feeling, and moral acting.

MORAL KNOWING

One important component of good character is *moral knowing.* But what is moral knowing?

Moral awareness. Moral knowing means, first of all, taking the time to think—to make a moral judgment about what is right and what is wrong. It is being aware that a particular situation involves moral issues.

One man describes how his parents helped him learn to do that: "Whenever I did something wrong, my parents didn't just demand that I stop my behavior. Instead, they almost always asked, 'How

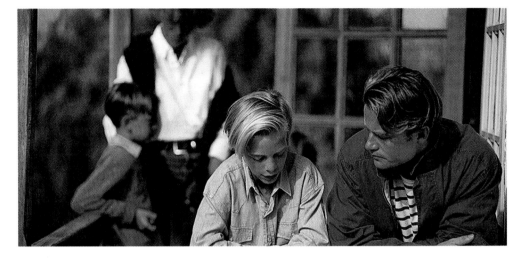

would you feel if someone did that to you?' That gave me a chance to reflect on whatever I did and how I'd like to have it done to me…. Now I try to stop and ask myself that question before I do something, rather than after the fact."[2]

Knowing moral values. The second element of moral knowing involves knowing those values that we use to distinguish right from wrong—values such as honesty, respect, kindness, compassion, courage, and responsibility.

Knowing moral values also involves understanding how they apply to various circumstances. What does responsibility mean when you see your best friend shoplifting? How do you show respect for your little brother who has Down's syndrome when people at the ballpark stare at him? What does respect mean on a date?

Perspective-taking. A third element of moral knowing is being able to understand someone else's point of view. Can you step into another person's shoes— and figure out how he or she might think or react or feel if you take a cer-

tain action? To respect other people and act according to their needs, you must first understand them.

Moral reasoning. The fourth element of moral knowing is moral reasoning. It helps us answer such questions as, Why should I study for my history exam? Why should I stand up for my little brother? Why should I volunteer to serve meals once a week at the local homeless shelter? Why should I call that girl I promised to call?

Why you do something can be just as important as what you do. We all know that people can do the right thing for the wrong reasons. As people develop and mature, they learn to distinguish between morally acceptable reasons for doing something and morally unacceptable reasons for doing it.

Some of the right reasons for doing things include showing respect for someone's worth as a person and treating others the way you would want to be treated.

Self-knowledge. A fifth aspect of moral knowing is self-knowledge. It includes such things as honestly assessing your attitudes and behavior, understanding your motives, being aware of your strengths and weaknesses, and knowing how to compensate for your weaknesses. This is perhaps the toughest aspect of moral knowing because it requires admitting your shortcomings and mistakes, rather than simply making excuses or trying to justify yourself.

Decision-making. Good decision-making depends on the previous five elements. Once you

- are aware that a situation demands a moral judgment,
- know which moral values apply to your situation,
- can take the perspective of others affected by the situation,
- are able to reason morally, and
- can assess your motives, strengths, and weaknesses,

then you are ready to decide what course of action is best in a given situation.

Good decision-making requires figuring out what your options are, determining their probable consequences for everyone affected by your actions, and then evaluating which option is best from both a moral and practical standpoint. The key question you need to answer here is this: Among those options that are morally acceptable, which are likely to have the best consequences for everyone involved?

These six elements—moral awareness, knowing moral values, perspective-taking, moral reasoning, self-knowledge, and decision-making—make up the moral knowing component of good character.

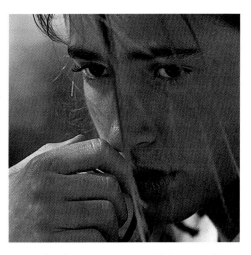

Just knowing what is right isn't always enough. A person must also care about what is right. That's a second important component of good character: *moral feeling.* Your moral emotions can help you do the right thing.

Melissa Whitaker, from chapter 1, cared about doing the right thing. When she said OK to Steve's request to see his house, she did it without thinking. But when she entered his house, she felt that she might have made the wrong decision. And her feelings were right.

The woman who returned the wallet because of guilty feelings from an earlier incident also cared about doing the right thing. She wanted to be honest, and her feelings reflected that.

Both Melissa and the woman not only knew the right thing, but they also cared about it. Moral feeling accompanied their moral knowing.

Conscience. It's important to understand that the feeling we're talking about is not simply your emotions. Rather it's an appreciation for what is right. That appreciation helps you put aside other feelings and gives you the desire to do what is right.

That's where conscience, one element of moral feeling, enters the picture. Your conscience can help you decide which emotions to act upon. You may feel like swearing at your teacher or having sex with someone or killing yourself. But your conscience warns you not to act out those feelings.

Conscience—the feeling of obligation to do what is right—plays an important part in moral behavior. Jiminy, the persistent cricket in the movie *Pinocchio*, was the little puppet's conscience. He instructed Pinocchio in what was right and wrong, and helped him feel obliged to make the right choice. Through hard experience Pinocchio learned the importance of listening to his conscience. As a result, he learned the meaning of true love and became a real boy.

A healthy conscience can help us resist temptation by making us feel guilty when we do something wrong—or sometimes even before we do it.

"Morality messed with me," admitted the young man after he stuffed the twenty dollars in his pocket. "Morality" was his conscience.

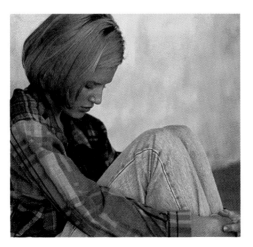

Self-respect. A second element of moral feeling, or the emotional side of character, is self-respect. How you feel about yourself can help you make the right choices and treat other people with respect.

Susan was a high school junior, a cheerleader, active in sports, and well-liked by her classmates. She also had a steady boyfriend. Then, just before her senior year, her family moved to another town. It was hard going at first. With no friends at the new high school she felt lost and alone—especially as a senior. Like most people, Susan wanted to be liked. She had been popular at her old school, but she didn't know what it took to be accepted by the new kids.

"I just have to find a friend," she told herself one night. "I'll do anything to fit in!"

Then Susan met Greg. He liked her.

"I fell in love," she said. "About three months into our relationship we started having sex. It was my first time. According to the kids at the new school, it seemed like the normal thing to do in a relationship."

Every time Susan and Greg had sex, she felt close to him.

"But when it was over, we got dressed, and I went home. There was no commitment, no assurance of tomorrow, and no feeling of true love from Greg, ever. When I woke up the next morning, I felt like a piece of trash. I knew in my heart that I was doing wrong. But I kept telling myself, 'This is OK. I'm giving love to someone.'

"The more I said that to myself, the worse it got, and the more I clung to Greg. I lost every bit of respect I'd ever had for myself." Susan told herself she needed the relationship because she had been so lonely before and felt more secure now. But eventually Greg broke up with her, and she began looking for love through sex in other relationships.[3]

Susan had gotten herself into a vicious cycle. Because of the way she felt about herself, she was willing to do things she didn't really think were right. But when she did them, it only diminished her self-respect and made her feel "like a piece of trash"—which in turn made it harder to follow her conscience when it told her *no*.

With a healthy self-respect, Susan would have depended more on what she knew was right and less on the approval of the other kids at school.

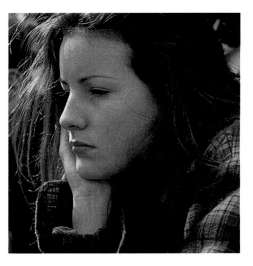

Empathy. Persons of good character are also capable of empathy, another element of moral feeling. Empathy is the capacity to feel what another person feels.

Ann Fowler, a high school senior and the oldest of seven children, learned empathy the hard way. Her mother developed cancer—a non-Hodgkin's lymphoma. She underwent chemotherapy and radiation treatments for two full years and was rarely available for her daughter when she needed her. As a result, Ann had no adult friend to turn to or attend school functions with her. She had to rely on herself and turned to her friends for support. She also had to give up her own time to help with her younger siblings. She became bitter.

"It wasn't fair," Ann says. "I felt anger toward her. I didn't believe she was sick."

But one day all that changed. Ann paid a surprise visit to her mother at the treatment center in Boston where she'd received a bone marrow transplant. She expected to find her mother smiling and happy, as she sounded in her letters and over the telephone. Instead, before she even walked in the room, Ann saw tears in her mother's eyes. For the first time she felt some of her mother's pain.

"I wished I could have done it for her," Ann says. "Seeing her that one day and seeing the tears in her eyes before I came into the room.... After that I decided to be unselfish and had a better life because of it."

Back home, Ann served her mother breakfast in bed, ran errands for her, did more chores around the house, and helped her brothers and sisters without being asked. Because of her empathy for her mother, Ann started putting her family first.

"I don't really feel like doing it, but I know my strength is a lot stronger than hers," she says.[4]

MORAL ACTING

Knowing what is right and wanting to do it are necessary ingredients of good character. But good character includes more than knowledge and feeling; it involves action—moral action. Unfortunately, *moral acting* doesn't always follow moral knowing and moral feeling. Sometimes it's hard to do what is right, even if you know what is right and want to do it. That is why the following are so important.

Moral competence. The first element of moral acting is moral competence. Moral competence consists of the skills and abilities you need to turn moral thinking and feeling into moral behavior.

Thousands of homeless people live on the streets of America. Segura Williams, then thirteen years old, along with his mother and nine sisters and brothers, lived in a tent in Los Angeles—in a campground for homeless people. Tired of being ignored by the city government, Segura pleaded his case alone before the Los Angeles City Council.

"We need so much help," Segura told the council, "and this problem is not going to go away unless we do something about it. We kids can make a difference. We want to help our families get out of here and into permanent houses."

The mayor of Los Angeles responded to Segura's plea and said he would visit the campsite in person to talk with the teenager and his friends.

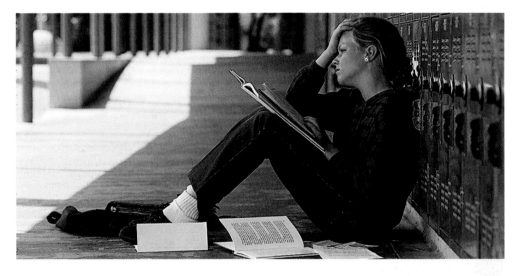

HOW MATURE ARE YOU?

HOW MATURE ARE YOU MENTALLY/INTELLECTUALLY?

- Do you know what it means to be courageous? respectful? responsible? self-controlled?
- Do you complete your homework and school assignments?
- Do you participate in class?
- Do you read great literature, or are you stuck reading comic books?
- Do you wait until the very last moment to complete school projects?
- Do you plan for future goals?

How Mature Are You Emotionally?

- Do you control your feelings when you don't get what you want?
- Do you call people names when you are angry?
- When a friend has a car and you don't, do you feel cheated?
- Can you discuss differences with your parents without yelling?
- If a person doesn't keep a promise, how do you respond?
- If your parents won't let you go out with your friends, do you control your emotions?
- If someone calls you a name, how do you respond?
- When things don't go your way, how do you respond?

How Mature Are You Morally?

- Do you stand up to your friends when they are putting someone down?
- Do you take things that don't belong to you?
- Have you ever taken money from your parents without their permission?
- Do you lie to your parents, teachers, friends, or others?
- Do you cheat on tests or copy friends' papers in school?
- If someone gives you too much money, do you give it back?
- Do you cut in lines?
- Do you rationalize, deny, or justify your friends' unhealthy behaviors?

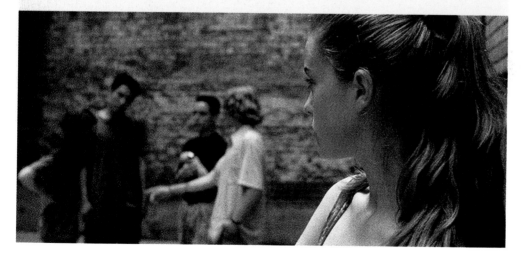

Segura organized Kids Helping Each Other to collect food, clothes, and money for the people who lived at the campground. He and his friends also started serving breakfast every day.

Segura Williams showed moral competence when he approached the city council with a plan of action and when he, with his friends, carried out the plan.[5]

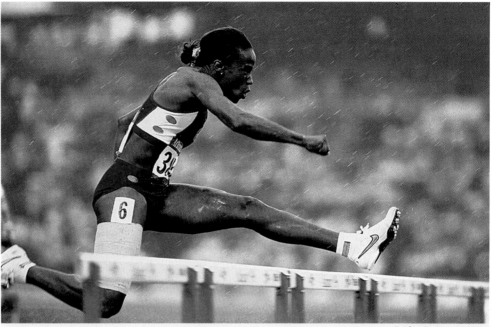

Jackie Joyner-Kersee

HOW MATURE ARE YOU SOCIALLY?

- Can you stand up to your friends when you know you are right, or do you go along with the crowd?
- Do you allow your friends to determine what type of behavior you will participate in?
- Will you put your health at risk simply to be liked by friends?
- Do you imitate your friends and use the same language and mannerisms they do to fit in with the group?
- What things will you do simply to be part of a group?

A person matures physically in about eleven or twelve years, but it takes hard work to mature and grow in the other developmental areas—mentally, emotionally, socially, morally. Sometimes we make mistakes and hurt other people, and even ourselves. Being mature requires us to keep trying even when we have made mistakes.

Anyone can be an adult. Immature adults remain self-satisfied in their inappropriate and unhealthy behaviors, such as cheating in school, engaging in premarital sex, using drugs, viewing pornography, or exploiting others sexually. Mature adults, unlike immature adults, stand a much better chance of becoming successful people and productive citizens.

Immature adults don't need to stay that way. They can turn their lives around and strive toward mature adulthood. But first they need to develop positive and healthy values for living.

Willpower. A second element of moral acting is willpower. Willpower is something track legend Jackie Joyner-Kersee knows a great deal about. Only a month before the 1996 Olympics in Atlanta, Georgia, Jackie pulled a hamstring at the U.S. Olympic trials. Despite her injury she qualified not only for the heptathlon, but also for the long jump.

At the Olympics she reaggravated her injury while running the hurdles portion of the heptathlon. Although in severe pain, Jackie completed the hurdles and started toward the next event of the heptathlon. She would have continued competing except that her coach and husband, Bobby Kersee, intervened.

A few days later she was still in pain but competed in the long jump. On her final jump she captured the bronze medal with a jump of more than twenty-two feet.

It was clear that Jackie's performances in both the Olympic trials and the Olympics were acts of willpower. After her bronze-medal long jump, Jackie told reporters, "Tonight is very special. I had to really work for this one. It really tested my determination. I had to be mentally tough."[6]

Jackie also said, "I want to be remembered as someone who gave 110 percent at all times. I never gave up tonight. I tried to improve and stay positive the whole time."[7]

Habit. A third element of moral acting is habit. People with good character have made a habit of choosing what is right. As former Secretary of Education William Bennett observes, people with good character "act truthfully, loyally, bravely, kindly and fairly without being much tempted by the opposite course."[8]

United States Senator Dan Coats of

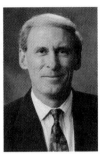

Senator Dan Coats

Indiana puts it this way: "Character cannot be summoned at the moment of crisis if it has been squandered by years of compromise and rationalization.... The only preparation for that one profound decision which can change a life, or even a nation, is those hundreds of half-conscious, self-defining, seemingly insignificant decisions made in private. Habit is the daily battleground of character."[9]

To help students form good character habits, the principal of an Atlanta high school requires the students to work in their communities for seventy-five hours before they graduate. Students in St. Louis and other cities also serve their communities while they attend high school. Such community service helps form good character because the students are developing habits of compassion and helpfulness, and learning to be good citizens.

To summarize, the three components of good character are moral knowing, moral feeling, and moral acting—

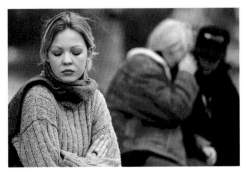

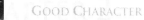

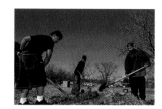

knowing the good, desiring the good, and doing the good. When we have good character, we are capable of judging what is right, we care deeply about what is right, and we consistently do what is right in our lives.

WHAT GOOD CHARACTER LOOKS LIKE

To do what's right when facing temptation, it's important to develop positive and healthy habits. Before we can do what's right, we need the ability to judge what's right. Also, we have to really care about it. Using the following scenarios, role play what good character would look like if you found yourself in each of these situations.

WHAT WOULD SELF-CONTROL LOOK LIKE IF...
- You're angry at your mom, and your friends ask you to go out drinking.
- A friend wants you to leave the restaurant without paying the bill.
- On a date, a boy makes sexual advances toward a girl.
- You're getting ready for a party and want to wear your favorite shirt, but your sister spilled something on it the last time she borrowed it.
- You hate playing basketball because you're not very good. Your dad asks you to play and teases you about your skill. You feel yourself getting angry and upset.

WHAT WOULD JUSTICE LOOK LIKE IF...
- You can't find your diary. You've looked everywhere. Your mother was in your room putting clothes away, and you think she may have taken it.
- Your friends are waiting for you at your locker. They are laughing and carrying on. You ask them what's so funny. They're making fun of a boy in math class because he wears thick-rimmed glasses, carries a ton of books, and wears his pants too short.
- One of your friends tells you that another buddy has been saying things behind your back. He also tells you that he's been saying things to your girlfriend.
- You've studied hard for your history final. You need an A to get an A in the class. A friend tells you prior to taking the exam that she hasn't studied and intends to cheat. Several days pass. You receive an A on the test, but your teacher announces that someone cheated on the test. If the person does not privately admit his/her mistake, everyone's grade in the class will be lowered.

- It's snowing and your school is closed for the day. Your friends want to go sledding. Your sister asks to come along.
- You're at a movie theater. The movie has ended, and you're leaving the theater with several friends. You run into Molly, a girl in your math class. Molly has a birth defect on her face. You both say hello. As soon as you continue on, your friends make fun of Molly.
- You dislike cats, but your sister loves them and receives one for her birthday. One afternoon you hear the kitten meowing at the door. Its fur is covered with burrs.

WHAT WOULD HUMILITY LOOK LIKE IF...

- You're trying out for cheerleading. It's time for you and your partner to be judged. After tryouts the new cheerleading squad is announced. Your partner makes it, but you don't. The judges want to know if anyone wants to see the scores.
- You and your friend are not speaking. You're angry at your friend for asking out a girl he knew you liked. You say things that you later regret.

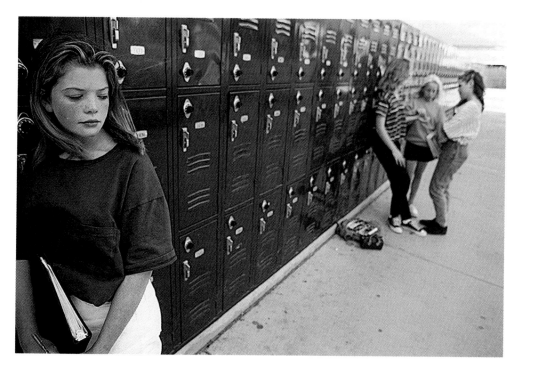

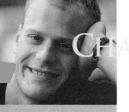
- You're having a hard time in algebra. The teacher tells the class that she'll remain after school for anyone who needs help. Several of your friends want you to go rollerblading after school.

WHAT WOULD HONESTY LOOK LIKE IF...

- You and your family are having breakfast at a restaurant. After the meal, your parents pay the bill and finish their coffee. You notice on the bill that the waitress didn't charge you enough for your meal.
- Several friends meet after school on Friday to decide what to do for the weekend. There's a big party Saturday evening. It's been decided that you should tell your parents you're spending the night at a friend's home, but instead you'll be at the all-night party.
- It's Saturday night, and you're out with a girl you really like. Lately, you've been pressured by friends to make sexual advances toward this girl. You know she likes you. You like and respect her too.

WHAT WOULD COURAGE LOOK LIKE IF...

- You're at an unsupervised party. Several friends are in the kitchen drinking and laughing. Also in the kitchen is a girl you like. Your friends ask you if you'd like a drink. Everyone is waiting for a response.
- After school you're supposed to finish a science lab. Friends want you to go to the mall. One friend gives you his lab work to copy so you can go to the mall. They continue to harass you.
- You overhear a group of friends talking about your neighbor. Your neighbor has a growth on her face. Friends are making fun of her appearance.

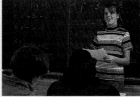

- You've been assigned to give your group's presentation. You dislike speaking in front of others. Part of the group's grade is based on the presentation.

WHAT WOULD RESPECT LOOK LIKE IF...

- You've just purchased a new CD and want to use your brother's CD player, but he is not around to ask.
- You need five dollars for school, and you see some money sticking out of your mom's purse.
- You suspect that your brother smokes cigarettes. You walk into his room to ask him a question, but he's not there. His backpack, however, is open on his desk.
- There is a rule at home that you don't agree with.
- A handwritten note has fallen out of your sister's purse.
- You've unexpectedly been given a low grade on your English paper. You find yourself talking rudely to your teacher.

- You promised a friend that you'd meet her after school, but later you remember that you have a session with your math tutor.
- While rushing into a convenience store you park your father's car in a handicap space. Upon returning you find a ticket on the car.
- You are over at a friend's house watching videos. Your friend's parents want to take the two of you out for dinner. You remember that you promised to take your younger sister ice skating.
- You have promised your mom to move the dining room furniture because the room is going to be painted. Your friends call and ask you to play a pickup game of football at the park.

VALUES AND GOOD CHARACTER

Not every action shows good character. That's because good character depends on moral values. Some actions are right; some are wrong. But what are moral values? To understand what moral values are, it might help to contrast them with both facts and preferences.

When we state a fact, we're stating something about the way things are. Here are some examples:
- The sky is cloudy today.
- I'm tired.
- Jim is over six feet tall.
- Amy pushed Jessica.

Moral values, on the other hand, tell us something about the way things *ought* to be—what we should and shouldn't do, even if we don't feel like it. We call these *core ethical values*.
- Be kind to others.
- Take only what belongs to you.
- Share with others.
- Wait for your turn.

Moral values also differ from preferences. When we talk about our preferences, we're talking about what we like and dislike.
- I really don't want to go out tonight.
- I'd rather have orange juice than lemonade.
- I like your outfit.
- This ride is great.

These preferences, or nonmoral values, do not carry obligation and do not involve right and wrong. People with sound moral feeling prefer moral values. But moral values go beyond mere preferences because they are morally binding. Under most circumstances, choosing orange juice over lemonade is neither morally good nor morally bad. Ethically speaking, we're free to choose either one. We're not free, however, to steal someone else's money or to treat animals cruelly. Many people choose to do those things, but we recognize that such choices are wrong.

Of course, people may disagree over certain values. Many Muslims and Jews, for example, believe it is wrong to eat pork. Similarly, some religious groups believe that it is wrong for men and women to associate with each other unless they are relatives.

Despite some differences, many ethical

values are recognized the world over. They are right and good whether or not a person realizes it. They are also consistent with the great moral principles found in many religions and cultures— such as the Golden Rule: "Do unto others as you would have others do unto you." These values include compassion, honesty, perseverance, courage, humility, responsibility, respect, and tolerance. We'll look at some of them now.

COMPASSION

Of all the values, compassion is the most human. The word itself literally means "to suffer with." Having compassion means that you understand the sufferings of others and are moved to help them.

You can often see compassion displayed after major disasters, such as earthquakes, floods, or hurricanes. After

Hurricane Andrew struck South Florida in August 1992, hundreds of volunteers from across the nation rushed in to provide food and other badly needed supplies. Many stayed for months, repairing and rebuilding people's homes.

You can also see compassion in less extreme circumstances, such as when neighbors or church members do yard work or home repairs for someone who is sick or disabled. Or when people volunteer at crisis pregnancy centers and open their homes to pregnant girls who need a place to stay. Or when someone with a million things to do stops and listens to a hurting friend.

Compassion is one of the greatest values.

HONESTY

Honesty is another important value. To understand how essential it is, think about times when people have treated you or a family member or a friend dishonestly. Have you ever had anything stolen? Have you ever been lied to or lied about? Has a family member or friend ever been cheated out of money? How did you feel when those things happened?

Honesty is vital to the well-being of any society. Imagine what would happen in a society where it was missing. Judges couldn't be counted on for justice. Police officers couldn't be counted on to protect innocent people. Food manufacturers couldn't be trusted to label their food products accurately. Pharmacy

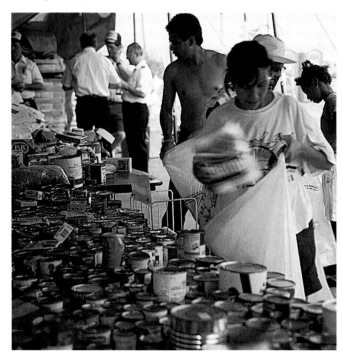

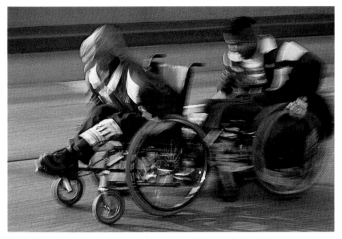

companies couldn't be trusted to report drug tests accurately. Building inspectors couldn't be trusted to ensure that builders used appropriate materials and methods.

In fact, we *can't* always count on people to be honest. That's why we have judges and police, along with hundreds of civilian and government "watchdog" organizations. But without honesty we could count on no one.

Perseverance

Another trait found in a person of good character is perseverance. Perseverance is the ability to keep doing something even if it's difficult or unpleasant. The story of Charla Ramsey and Sacajuwea Hunter illustrates this. These two girls met in school through their common interest in sports and persevered in spite of great odds.

At fourteen, Saca became the youngest member of the U.S. Olympic team and was rated as the fourth fastest person in the world in her event: long-distance wheelchair racing. She worked hard to achieve those goals, especially since both of her legs were amputated when she was a baby. Her mother had placed her in a tub of scalding water and burned her legs so badly that they could not be saved. The court took Saca from her mother, and another family later adopted her.

Charla Ramsey was born with spina bifida: her spinal column was malformed. But in 1982, at age thirteen, she became the youngest person to be accepted on the U.S. wheelchair racing team and went on to compete internationally, using a wheelchair built for racing. In 1992 Charla won the one-hundred-meter race at the World Championship Games in Paris. She became the fastest in the world in that event.[10]

Both Saca and Charla demonstrated perseverance and self-discipline to overcome their disabilities.

Hope is a close ally of perseverance. Do you remember Segura Williams, who lived with his family in a campground for the homeless in Los Angeles? Thirteen-year-old Segura approached the city council with a plan to help the homeless; influenced the mayor to visit the campground; rallied other kids to collect food, clothes, and money; and succeeded in helping the families in his campground. Segura didn't let his homelessness discourage him. He had hope and perseverance.

You may never encounter challenges like the ones Charla, Saca, and Segura faced. But sooner or later all of us will face problems that can only be solved with persistence and determination.

COURAGE

Courage is another character trait that doesn't come easily. People with courage do what's right even if it is frightening or dangerous. We all know about people who were willing to sacrifice their lives because of what they knew was right. Mother Teresa and Mahatma Gandhi are two well-known examples.

But courage is not just for adults. Five-year-old Rocky Lyons, son of football player Marty Lyons, demonstrated great courage—and perseverance—when he overcame his fear and saved his mother's life. Rocky and his mother were coming home from a dinner with friends. Suddenly, the Ford pickup his mother was driving hit a pothole, veered off the road, hit the side of a bridge, and flipped over and over down the side of a hill, crushing the roof. The little boy slept through the ordeal and woke up when the truck stopped.

Rocky could tell that his mother was badly hurt. One shoulder was almost ripped off, the other was crushed, and there was so much blood in her eyes that she couldn't see.

"We've got to get you up the hill. We've got to get you to a hospital, Mama," he told her calmly, despite his fear of what could happen if they didn't make it.

She tried to dig her fingers in the dirt and pull herself up the hill, but she couldn't because she had no strength in her arms. Rocky got behind her and tried to push her, but she still couldn't make it. Finally, he remembered *The Little Engine That Could*, the story his mother had read to him again and again when he was little. Whenever he thought he couldn't do something, she would remind him of the little train.

"Mama, think about the train," Rocky told his mother now. "I think I can…I think I can…I think I can…I think I can."

So she kept thinking she could until he had helped her up the hill to the side of the road. Two cars passed without stopping. Rocky was afraid for his mom. Yet, far from being immobilized by his fears, he grabbed his mother's hand, and they started walking. Just then another car stopped and took them to a hospital.

Because of Rocky's courage and determination, his mother lived. And despite the doctors' predictions that she would never use her arms, she was fine a year after the accident.[11]

RESPONSIBILITY

At the heart of responsibility is doing what you agree or commit to doing. Being responsible means being the kind of person that others can rely on—you can be trusted with new tasks and freedoms. New tasks might include such things as running errands with the car or watching a younger brother or sister when your parents have to go somewhere. New freedoms might include

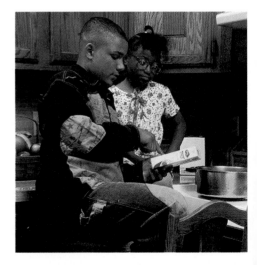

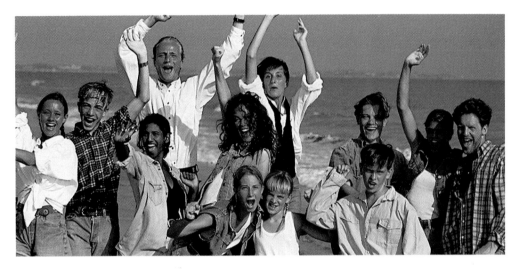

going on the senior beach trip or on an overnight outing with friends.

But being responsible means more than being reliable. It also means that you feel a sense of obligation for the welfare of others. Not only do you avoid actions that could hurt people, but you become involved in actively helping them. In fact, responsibility is closely related to compassion, and it often springs from empathy.

That is clear from Ann Fowler's story, mentioned earlier in this chapter. When Ann saw her mother's suffering, she began taking responsibility for the welfare of her mother and siblings. She no longer did just what she had to or what she was asked to do, but she also looked for new ways to help.

Respect

Like responsibility, respect covers a lot of territory. Literally, the word means "to look back at" or "consider." It implies that the person or object you're looking at is worth more than a hasty glance—that the person or object is worth treating with care.

Although this comes close to describing the essence of respect, the term has many shades of meaning, mostly depending on the recipient of your respect. For example, when you respect friends or peers, you value them. You see them as having worth. As a result, you treat them with consideration and avoid doing things that would hurt them in any way. It also means treating them the way you would want to be treated.

On the other hand, when you respect parents or teachers—or anyone else in a position of authority—you treat them with consideration and honor. That includes obeying them in their proper sphere of authority and addressing them courteously, instead of being rude.

But respect goes far beyond the treatment of other people. All of us, for example, should respect the laws where we live, whether at home, at school, in a dorm, or in the community. We should also respect the environment.

Tolerance

Tolerance enables us to respect people even when they differ with us on impor-

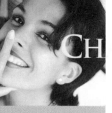

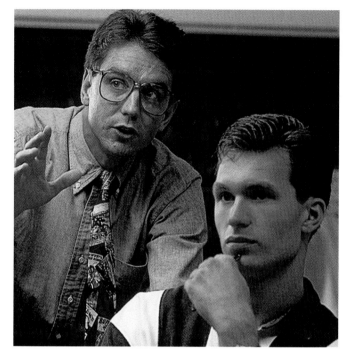

grade students take part in an eight-week course called Facing History and Ourselves. They study the Nazi Holocaust and how people around the world continue to be prejudiced and mistreat each other. One of the questions the students consider is, "How could the Holocaust happen?" They keep track of their thoughts and feelings in journals. One girl wrote at the end of the course:

I'm glad this unit was taught to us, and especially to me. At the beginning I have to admit I was prejudiced against Jews and was glad they were killed. I know this is awful, especially if that is your religion. Then you and the class discussions proved to me I was wrong! Jewish is just like me and other people.[12]

Like Sean and Maurice in Ireland, this middle-school girl learned tolerance—and respect—for people who are different from her.

tant topics. It's an attitude that values others despite our differences.

For her class in creative writing for children, Nicki, a college student, wrote a story that illustrated the value of tolerance. Since Nicki was Irish and grew up in Ireland, her story depicted the prejudice that exists between Protestants and Catholics there.

Two Irish boys—Maurice, a Catholic, and Sean, a Protestant—lived in different neighborhoods. Because of religious prejudice, Maurice and Sean were taught to hate each other. One day they were playing in a community pool when Maurice, who couldn't swim, started to drown. Sean saved his life. Concern for someone in danger overcame religious differences. The boys became friends and tried to convince the adults in their lives that it was good to be friends, regardless of a person's religion.

In Brookline, Massachusetts, eighth-

Robert Coles, Harvard child psychiatrist and author of *The Moral Life of Children*, investigated the moral lives of young people. He interviewed selected teachers and students at two public high schools, George Washington Carver in Atlanta and Highland Park near Chicago, and at a private boarding school, St. Paul's, near Concord, New Hampshire. He was interested in teachers who were "qualified to judge character" and students who, in the teachers' opinions, possessed "character" or "high character." He told the students he wanted to find out what character meant to them.

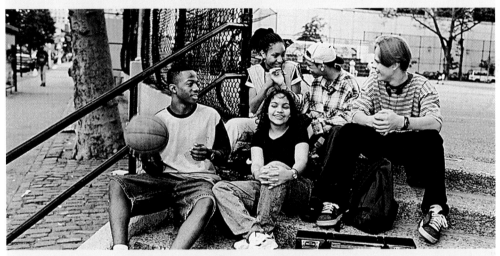

Some students believed that how a person responds to others is important. One young man described his own experience: "I tend to be a private person. I like to take long walks by myself. At times I don't want company; I want to hold on to my individuality. But I like to be with others, too. I like to be a friend. I'd like to think that if someone were in trouble, he'd turn to me, and I'd be there, and I'd put that person's trouble above my needs, including taking a solitary walk!"[13]

The students at St. Paul's produced a list of the traits they thought made up character:
- a person who sticks to a set of principles;
- a person who can risk unpopularity, yet is commanding enough to gain the respect of others;
- a person who has the courage to be himself or herself;
- a person who is open-minded, who plays fair with others, who doesn't lie and cheat and deceive himself or herself.[14]

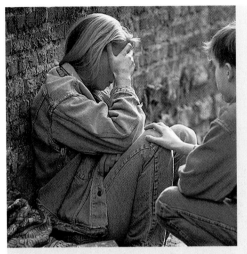

One student thought that "there are reasons we end up being one kind of person or another kind of person, but when you actually become that person (when you're nice to others most of the time), then that's a true achievement. A lot of people don't become nice, and it's no excuse to say you had a bad childhood or you never had the right luck. I think you have to take your troubles and overcome them!"[15]

Another student thought that character was "what you decide to do for others, not just for yourself."[16]

For this group of students at St. Paul's, character meant "a quality of mind and heart one struggles for, at times with a bit more success than at others."[17]

At Highland Park High School north of Chicago, Dr. Coles invited a similar discussion.

Some of the students said that character had to do with popularity. But two disagreed: "Character has to do with honesty. You can be popular, and have a shrink's seal of approval, but not have character!"[18]

These students also discussed whether a person's financial status affected character. One student offered this opinion: "It's easier to be generous if you've got a lot behind you!"[19]

But another student countered, "I know some kids…from pretty poor families, compared to others; their fathers just get by, make a living. And they would give you the shirt off their backs, those kids: that's character. And they wouldn't go talking about what they've done, bragging and showing off—that's character!

"Some people," she continued, "they know how to play up to the teachers, and they get a big reputation, but what's the truth about them? What are they like when no one is looking, and what are they like when no one is listening?"[20]

Together the students at Highland Park concluded that the "way-down-deep truth" of a person was what counted. And that truth, which for them meant character, was tested when sickness, financial problems, or a disaster hit.[21]

The students suggested that literature offered a way to understand character. For example, in *To Kill a Mockingbird* Atticus possessed character: "He was open-minded, stood up for what he believed, no matter the risks and costs, and so was a 'moral man.'" In Shakespeare's *Macbeth*, Lady Macbeth was a "bad person," a "bad character."[22]

One young woman, the least talkative, added that "character meant being kind and good, even when there was no one to reward you for being kind and good."[23]

The students agreed: "You are the way you act—in the long run."[24]

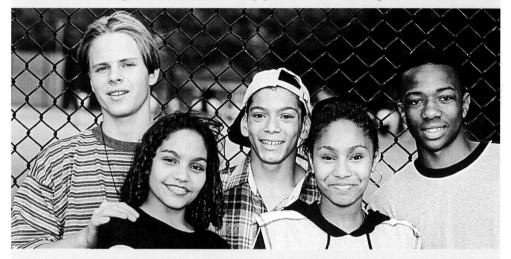

At Atlanta's George Washington Carver High School, the principal told Dr. Coles: "Character is something you have to build…every day…. Character means discipline and hard work and looking to the future and getting there!"[25]

The students at Carver offered a slightly different perspective. They said they were committed to hard work and finding jobs, to being strong parents—and they believed that commitment was connected to character.

But, they felt, as one put it, "a lot of us, even here, with the principal and the teachers bearing down every minute on us, have trouble reading and writing. We're not going to college, most of us. We're going to try to get a job and hold on to it! It takes character, I think, to do that—not take the easy way out and drink or use drugs or say the white man is on our backs, so what the devil can we do! To me, character is being stubborn. It's staying in there—it's getting out of a hole and breathing the fresh air and not falling down any more."[26]

"It's not only getting there," another said; "it's *how* you get there. If you have character, that means you keep trying, no matter how hard it is, and you don't lose your soul while you're doing that. You have to say to yourself, 'I'll go so far and no farther.' You have to draw the line, and if you do, and you can hold to it, you've got character."[27]

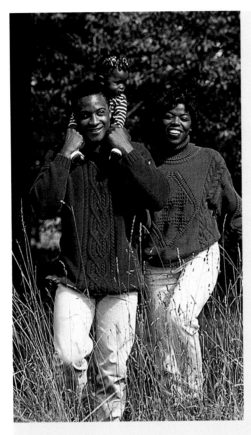

"Building" oneself into "a stronger person" and getting "on the map" were important to the Atlanta students. For them that involved getting jobs at places like auto repair shops, television and radio repair shops, dry-cleaning shops, and the big airport.

They agreed that "if you get one of those jobs, and you hold on to it; if you get yourself a girlfriend or a boyfriend, and they become a wife or a husband, and you become a father or a mother, and you 'stay with it,' and are good to your family, earn them a living, take care of them; if you remain loyal to your church and pray to God when you're weak; if you don't forget your people and try to lend a hand to the ones who didn't make it, who stumbled and fell and are hurt and sad and who are wondering what the point of it all is, and maybe have done wrong, done it too many times—if all that is 'inscribed on your soul,' then, by God, you have character, and it's important to say 'by God,' because it's 'His grace that does things.' "[28]

The Atlanta students didn't think "good manners" were at all superficial. As one expressed it, "They tell of something very deep down."[29]

Another student said, "You can tell a person by how he speaks to you. If he's respectful, then he's good; if he gives you the shoulder, then he's bad."[30]

"We all stray," voiced one young woman. "But if we try hard not to keep repeating ourselves, and if we're not afraid to learn from our mistakes, and if we're willing to work hard, and sacrifice, then we have character."[31]

One of the teachers from George Washington Carver High School expressed her opinion on character this way: "I don't think character is the property of the lucky and the smart and the successful, no sir. But to me, character means an active person, who is ready to face the world and make a mark on it.... Never be lazy."[32]

WHY IS GOOD CHARACTER SO IMPORTANT?

As the Greek philosopher Heraclitus has said, "Character is destiny." This is true in many ways; our character affects us, our friends, our families, our acquaintances, and our entire society.

How Our Character Affects Us

Joe was one young man whose character affected both him and the people around him. In his teen years he'd had sex with a lot of girls. In doing so, he contracted a sexually transmitted disease (STD). Eventually he settled down, found a good job, and married a young woman named Cheryl. A year later Joe and Cheryl had a baby boy. They named him Tommy. Because of Joe's STD, which he had passed on to his wife, Tommy was born blind.[33]

As a teenager, Joe put his own pleasure first—and ended up sacrificing the health of his wife and his child. His character thus affected his future as a husband and a father in ways he never imagined. Once you learn and commit to practicing good character, however, you can become a better friend, a better spouse, a better parent, and a better citizen.

Having good character will also help you succeed in your career. To survive as an adult in today's world, you must know how to work (responsibility), how to arrive at your job on time (self-discipline and responsibility), how to get along with your coworkers and others (honesty, respect, responsibility, compassion, and humility), how to stick with a task until you've finished it (perseverance and self-discipline), and how

to respect legitimate authority.

Self-discipline is especially important. To cope with the demands of modern life you need an adequate dose of self-discipline. Discipline, a mark of good character, is the secret behind a beautiful symphony, a gold-medal Olympic athlete, a championship football team, a profitable business, or a successful school.

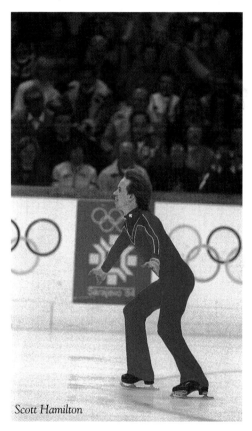

Scott Hamilton

According to pollster Daniel Yankelovich, what we consider valuable has changed over time. Overall, we place a higher value now on such things as personal choice, self-expression, self-realization, and individualism; and less value on such things as moral obligation, sacrifice as a moral good, social

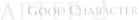

conformity, respectability, and following rules. We also place less value on being correct and restraining ourselves when it comes to physical pleasure and sexuality.[34]

HOW OUR CHARACTER AFFECTS OTHERS

In the previous section, we saw that your character will determine what kind of a friend, spouse, parent, and citizen you will be. Since each of these roles involves other people, the kind of character you exhibit will have a profound effect on other people—and ultimately on society itself.

The effect of character on society is clearly visible in statistics from the last thirty to forty years. These figures

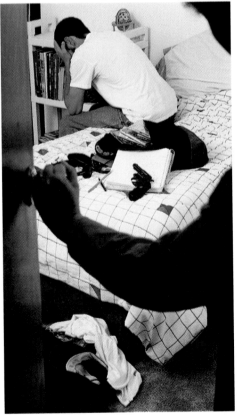

indicate a steep decline in the character of Americans. Here are some of these statistics:

- From 1960 to 1992, violent crimes increased more than 500 percent, and total crimes increased more than 300 percent. During the same period America's population grew only 41 percent. The rate of violent crime in the United States is worse than in any other industrialized country.[35] What's more, America's children make up the fastest growing segment of the criminal population.[36] The Federal Bureau of Investigation (FBI) reports a four-fold increase in juvenile arrests from 1965 to 1990. The FBI figures reflect crime increases not only among disadvantaged minority youth, but among youth from all races, lifestyles, and social classes.[37]

- Births out of wedlock have soared. In 1960 the number of unmarried women giving birth while unmarried was about one in twenty. By the early nineties that number had increased to about one in three.[38] That's not counting the number of pregnancies terminated by abortion. The Alan Guttmacher Institute reports that sexual activity among adolescents produces about one million pregnancies each year, a third of which end in abortions.[39]

- The divorce rate in America is about double what it was in the early 1960s. Starting from a low of fewer than ten divorces per one thousand marriages annually, it climbed to a high of twenty-three per one thousand before declining slightly to about twenty-one per thousand in the early 1990s. Over the same time period, the number of marriages per thousand unmarried women declined from about seventy-four to fifty-four.[40] At these rates, almost half of all marriages can be expected to end in divorce.

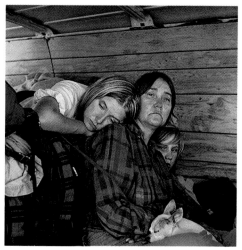

- The number of children who live with only one parent has more than tripled in the past thirty years. About 90 percent of such households do not have a father. Seventy-three percent of children who live with only one parent will experience poverty sometime while they are young, compared to 20 percent of children living with two parents. Fewer than 60 percent of today's children live with their married, biological parents.
- According to the Centers for Disease Control (CDC), acquired immune deficiency syndrome (AIDS) is the number one killer of people ages twenty-five to forty-four.[41] It's the sixth leading cause of death among teenagers and young adults ages fifteen to twenty-four. In 1993, it killed more young people

than any other infectious disease.[42] AIDS is also the seventh leading cause of death among children ages one to four.[43]
- Students' scores on the Scholastic Aptitude Test (SAT) have fallen almost eighty points since the 1960s. At the same time, spending on education has risen significantly. But so has the amount of time students spend watching TV.[44] Recent comparisons show that American students spend far more time watching television and far less time doing homework than students in other nations.[45] Many writers have pointed out that a democratic, technologically advanced society cannot survive for long if its citizens are uneducated and illiterate. Recently the Educational Testing Service, which administers the SAT, has called for a major change in American attitudes to reverse these trends.[46]

Of the above items, perhaps the two most ominous ones concern births outside of marriage, and divorce. As researcher Barbara Dafoe Whitehead concludes in a cover story for *The Atlantic Monthly*, "Growing up in an intact two-parent family is an important source of advantage for American children."[47] From her research she cites three "structural constants" that are found in intact, or whole, families:

Economics. Children in intact families typically share in the income produced by two adults. Today, in fact, two-parent families are needed more instead of less, because more families need both incomes to afford adequate food, housing, and medical insurance.

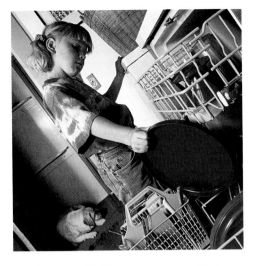

Authority. Children are more likely to find a stable authority structure in intact families, whereas a family that breaks up usually disturbs the proven boundaries of authority. Children are often expected to grow up quickly and act like mature adults, making decisions and accepting responsibilities that normally belong to parents. That frees the parents to deal with the emotional problems that result from their failed marriage. Without boundaries, everyone makes up his or her own rules. Children then lose the opportunity to test boundaries and discover what works and what doesn't on the way to developing their character.

Household personnel. Children in intact families do not suffer from a disturbed sense of peace or security because of new adults entering the household. In a disrupted family, stepparents and boyfriends or girlfriends may represent a threat to the well-being and security of the children.[48]

Cornell University psychologist Urie Bronfenbrenner points out that even when such things as family income are taken into account, children growing up in single-parent families are "at greater risk for experiencing a variety of behavioral and educational problems, including extremes of hyperactivity and withdrawal, lack of attentiveness in the classroom, difficulty in deferring gratification, impaired academic achievement, school misbehavior, absenteeism, dropping out, involvement in socially alienated peer groups, and especially the so-called 'teenage syndrome' of behaviors that tend to hang together—smoking, drinking, early and frequent sexual experience, and, in the more extreme cases, drugs, suicide, vandalism, violence and criminal acts."[49]

LOOKING TO THE FUTURE

Most of these statistics reveal how the absence of good character affects you in your current roles as family member, student, and friend—and in your future roles as spouse, parent, employee, citizen, and member of a community. Since behavior is a matter of choice, the choices you make today determine how you live now, as well as in the future.

But in recent years we've seen a growing concern about the decline of character in our society. As Congressman J. C. Watts of Oklahoma said, people often think that "the only thing right is to get by and the only thing wrong is to get caught."[50] The problem is that

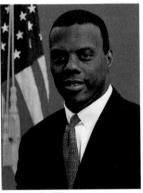

Rep. J. C. Watts

the things we get away with affect other people, and what we are in private can come out in public.

That's why character matters.

GOOD CHARACTER AS A LIFELONG PURSUIT

Developing good character is a lifelong task. When young people learn positive values such as honesty, helpfulness, kindness, love, being a good friend, and taking responsibility for their own actions, they are more likely to choose good actions over bad as they mature.

But young people who lack good character can still learn positive behaviors and attitudes. As psychologist and educator Tom Lickona writes, "Even if kids have not been given love in their homes, they can learn to give love to others who need it—and be surprised at the love that will come back to them…. The kind of love that helps them develop a positive self-concept. A sense of their worth. An inner strength."[51]

That inner strength is the substance of good character.

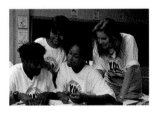

Throughout our lives the choices we make and the habits we forge shape our character. Of course, even people with excellent character will sometimes miss the mark. But since developing character is a lifelong pursuit, the more we lead a moral life, the more our thinking and feeling will get behind our action. There's no better satisfaction than a life well lived. Conversely, there's no worse pain than a life filled with bad choices.

EXAMINING YOUR OWN CHARACTER TRAITS

In the following pages you will have an opportunity to examine your character traits as a student, friend, son or daughter, club member, or athletic team member.

Read each statement in the tables below. On a separate sheet of paper write down the number from the column that best describes how often your behavior is consistent with the statement. After you do that for every statement in a given table, add up the numbers you've written down. The total is your overall rating for the character trait printed at the top of the table.

After you've taken this survey, encourage someone you know and trust—for example, a coach, friend, or roommate—to take the survey and evaluate your character. See how your answers compare. Discuss the results.

A score of 25–30 for a given table indicates that you usually exemplify that particular character trait. Congratulations! Keep up the good work. A score of 20–24 indicates that you are doing well but there is room for improvement. Developing positive habits requires perseverance. A score of 10–19 suggests that you need to improve your character. It will take self-control and determination to do so, but good character is never out of reach.

Throughout this book you'll find numerous suggestions for helping you improve your character.

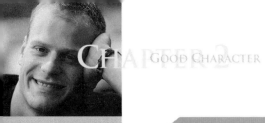

HONESTY	ALWAYS	SOMETIMES	NEVER
1. Report life-threatening and unhealthy behaviors to school administrators	3	2	1
2. Tell the truth to teachers	3	2	1
3. Cheat on tests or copy someone else's report	1	2	3
4. Occasionally shoplift	1	2	3
5. Tell the truth to parents	3	2	1
6. Tell the truth to friends	3	2	1
7. Exaggerate about accomplishments	1	2	3
8. Cover things up when you make a mistake	1	2	3
9. Promise to do things and then "forget"	1	2	3
10. Lie to others	1	2	3

Your overall Honesty rating: _____

RESPECT	ALWAYS	SOMETIMES	NEVER
1. Honor family and school rules	3	2	1
2. Read other people's private letters, diaries, etc.	1	2	3
3. Talk back to teachers, parents, or authority figures	1	2	3
4. Make fun of or talk back to elders	1	2	3
5. Interrupt or barge in on others	1	2	3
6. Treat others as if they don't matter	1	2	3
7. Use things without permission and/or never return borrowed items	1	2	3
8. Disrespect your body by using drugs or alcohol	1	2	3
9. Spread lies or gossip about others	1	2	3
10. Show obedience to parents and teachers	3	2	1

Your overall Respect rating: _____

COURAGE	ALWAYS	SOMETIMES	NEVER
1. Avoid doing things for fear of failing	1	2	3
2. Stand up for things you believe in	3	2	1
3. Afraid to admit mistakes	1	2	3
4. Do what everyone else does even if it is wrong	1	2	3
5. Do the easy thing and not the right thing	1	2	3
6. Be courageous even when others laugh at you	3	2	1
7. Confront others when they hurt someone	3	2	1
8. Refuse to drink, smoke, or use drugs	3	2	1
9. Able to ask for help when needed	3	2	1
10. Give up and quit when things go wrong	1	2	3

Your overall Courage rating: _____

SELF-DISCIPLINE	ALWAYS	SOMETIMES	NEVER
1. Overdo things or let yourself become too lazy	1	2	3
2. Lose control when you feel hurt or angry	1	2	3
3. Choose what is right in life	3	2	1
4. Procrastinate when you have a task to complete	1	2	3
5. Do whatever you feel like doing	1	2	3
6. Disregard rules at home and in school	1	2	3
7. Behave well only when you are being watched	1	2	3
8. Control your feelings when angry at a family member	3	2	1
9. Speak and act calmly when someone has angered you	3	2	1
10. Resist negative peer pressure	3	2	1

Your overall Self-Discipline rating: _____

JUSTICE	ALWAYS	SOMETIMES	NEVER
1. Talk behind someone else's back	1	2	3
2. Accuse someone before hearing his/her side of the story	1	2	3
3. Avoid getting involved if someone is getting hurt	1	2	3
4. Try to get away with things that are wrong	1	2	3
5. Treat people differently because of how they look	1	2	3
6. Share fairly with others	3	2	1
7. Look for the truth by investigating things for yourself	3	2	1
8. See people as individuals and not objects	3	2	1
9. Stand up for one's rights and the rights of others	3	2	1
10. Reward someone or recognize when someone is doing something right	3	2	1

Your overall Justice rating: _____

HUMILITY	ALWAYS	SOMETIMES	NEVER
1. Consider yourself more important than other people	1	2	3
2. Criticize others	1	2	3
3. Learn from your mistakes	3	2	1
4. Boast about your accomplishments	1	2	3
5. Do things only to impress others	1	2	3
6. Ask for help when needed	3	2	1
7. Respect what each person contributes	3	2	1
8. Focus on your growth and not on the faults of others	3	2	1
9. Worry about what others think about you	1	2	3
10. Expect yourself and others to be perfect	1	2	3

Your overall Humility rating: _____

RESPONSIBILITY	ALWAYS	SOMETIMES	NEVER
1. Teachers, parents, and coaches can depend on you	3	2	1
2. Accept correction when you do things wrong	3	2	1
3. Keep agreements and promises	3	2	1
4. Make excuses to get off the hook	1	2	3
5. Do things to the best of your ability	3	2	1
6. Agree to do things that are beyond your ability	1	2	3
7. Treat everything like a joke or a game	1	2	3
8. Complete household chores and school assignments	3	2	1
9. Look after younger siblings	3	2	1
10. Get to places on time	3	2	1

Your overall Responsibility rating: _____

KINDNESS	ALWAYS	SOMETIMES	NEVER
1. Concerned about the welfare of family members and friends	3	2	1
2. Show love to a sad friend or family member	3	2	1
3. Think of things that would make others happy	3	2	1
4. Resist the temptation to be cruel to a family member	3	2	1
5. Neglect one's pets and hurt animals	1	2	3
6. Tease and play tricks on someone you don't like	1	2	3
7. Ignore or ridicule someone who is different	1	2	3
8. Expect something in return for your help	1	2	3
9. Be kind only to those who are kind to you	1	2	3
10. Keep reminding others of how much you have helped or given	1	2	3

Your overall Kindness rating: _____

1. How did you do on the self-evaluation character survey? Building character takes time, perseverance, and hard work. Discuss the difficulties and rewards of improving your character.

2. Practicing the Golden Rule means that you "do unto others as you would have others do unto you." Do couples who engage in premarital sex break the Golden Rule? Is it ever necessary to take serious risks with your own or another person's physical, emotional, or spiritual welfare? Does premarital sex involve such risks?

3. Theodore Roosevelt is quoted at the beginning of this chapter: "To educate a person in mind and not in morals is to educate a menace to society." Is he right? What does this quote mean?

4. Congressman J. C. Watts of Oklahoma said people often think that "the only thing right is to get by and the only thing wrong is to get caught." Give some examples that illustrate this point.

5. In this chapter you learned that character, good and bad, affects every area of your life. Give some examples of how good and bad character can affect you, your family, your friends, and your future.

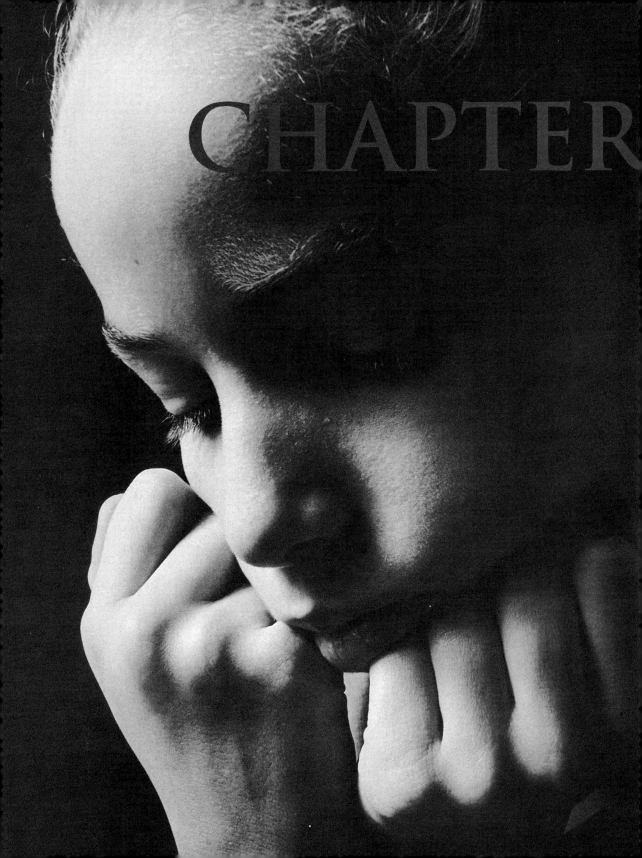

CHAPTER

3

CHARACTER AND SEXUALITY

-Rep. J. C. Watts

One cold Saturday in January 1995 Tanya Fontaine, a high school junior, met nineteen-year-old Bryan Nikolaj. They were piled into a car with a group of their friends on the way to the mall. To Tanya, Bryan's stocky build made him look like a pro-football linebacker. She smiled shyly at him. He smiled back.

Bryan was visiting his sisters and his divorced father in Manchester, New Hampshire. More than a year earlier, he had dropped out of school. Since then he had worked at odd jobs.

Tanya came from a different world. She lived at home with her parents, attended church each week, and was a good student. But she was attracted to Bryan's wild and independent spirit, and soon fell in love with him. She was certain her love would settle him down.

The two teenagers had sex after only a few dates. Then Tanya missed her period. The store-bought pregnancy test registered positive.

Tanya was nervous when she told Bryan, but his response, although a little slow in coming, put her at ease. "If you have the baby, I'll help you through it."

She hoped they would get married soon after the baby was born.

Tanya saw Bryan as her future husband, while her parents, shocked by the news, saw him as an irresponsible boy without goals or ambition.

"Life gets tougher as you get older," Tanya's mother told her. "Hard-working men like your father are difficult to find."

Tanya was too excited about starting her own life to heed her mother's warning. With help from a job as a waitress, she rented a small apartment.

Bryan accepted a job offer in her father's roofing business but quit after two days saying he was afraid of heights. He never stayed at a job for more than a few days, but continued to live at Tanya's apartment and use her car.

Tanya hoped Bryan would settle down after he saw the baby. When she went into labor in September, Bryan appeared at the hospital, then left for a sandwich. He returned, then left, and finally came back to watch the birth of the baby.

Tanya hoped Bryan would remain with her now that the baby, Ari, had arrived. But the young man was overcome by the baby's cries for food, clean diapers, and love. His time at the apartment became less frequent. After several months of feeling frustrated, Tanya finally asked Bryan to move out.

Tanya takes in about $270 a week from working as a waitress and a housekeeper. She can't move back with her parents. When necessary, they'll help her with the finances, but they've told her she's on her own. She gets no support from Bryan.

"I wish I could turn back the clock and be part of a family again," Tanya says. "I thought I knew what I was doing when I had sex. I didn't think I'd end up so alone."[1]

Sexuality, like so many other areas in our lives, involves character; and character has real-world consequences.

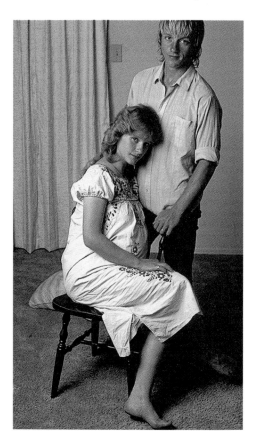

Tanya and Bryan did not consider how their actions would impact their future. When it was time for Bryan to take responsibility as a father, he felt overwhelmed and shirked his duty; he lacked the perseverance to stay on a job and thus failed to provide child support. Tanya was forced to take two jobs to support herself and her new son.

Many people don't realize that sexuality involves character. In this chapter and the three that follow, you will see just how crucial character is in sexual and romantic relationships. The remainder of this chapter looks at some of the benefits of good character, as well as some of the ways people hurt each other and themselves when they exhibit bad character. Chapters 4, 5, and 6 then focus on three particularly important topics: sexually transmitted disease (STD), pregnancy, and the emotional consequences of unmarried sex.

GOOD CHARACTER IN ROMANTIC RELATIONSHIPS

Any relationship benefits from good character. But because romantic relationships typically involve greater intimacy than other relationships, the benefits of good character for romantic relationships are especially valuable. Here are a few of those benefits:

- **When both of you possess good character, you can count on each other to be faithful and honest.** You don't have to worry about whether your partner is cheating on you or trying to conceal something from you. And your partner doesn't have to worry about you. The two of you will be less likely to be anxious when you're apart, and your relationship is less likely to be hindered by suspicion.

- **When both of you possess good character, you don't have to impress each other.** You can be confident that your partner loves you for who you are—and not for what you have or what you can give. You don't have to wonder if your partner likes you simply because you are popular or physically attractive or have a car or are willing to have sex. And your partner doesn't have to wonder about you. When you are together, you can relax and be yourselves because you're free from the burden of "performing" for each other.
- **When both of you possess good character, you can relax your defenses.** Just as you don't have to impress each other, you also don't have to worry about being manipulated.
- **When both of you possess good character, you will each have someone with whom you can talk and share your feelings.** As was mentioned in chapter 2, good character

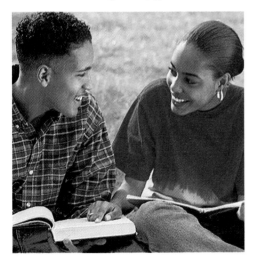

involves the ability not only to understand another person's point of view, but also to feel what that person feels. That doesn't mean that your partner will always agree with you—or that you should always agree with your partner. But it does mean that you have someone who will take you seriously and not brush you off or ridicule you. Equally important, you can be sure that your partner will never reveal your secrets or use them against you.

- **When both of you possess good character, you can count on one another to keep your word.** If, for example, your partner agrees to meet you somewhere, you know that your partner will be there. If the two of you agree to go on a date, you know that your partner won't cancel on you if something "better" comes along. If your partner agrees to help you with a difficult or boring task, you can be sure you'll get help.

An important part of exercising good character in your romantic relationships is abstaining from sex until marriage and remaining monogamous thereafter. Of course, there's more to good character than abstaining from sex before marriage, but even this one thing brings numerous rewards. In particular you will enjoy many freedoms that you might otherwise lose or miss. These include:

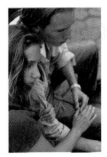

- **Freedom from pregnancy and all that it entails (premature parenting, adoption, abortion).** If a couple has a sexual relationship, the girl may become

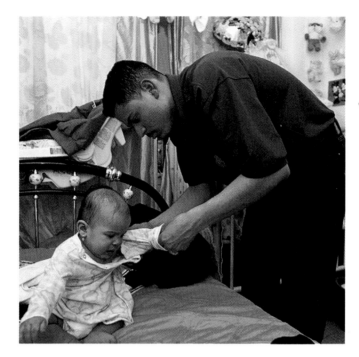

pregnant. If that occurs, the couple must decide either to have the baby or to abort. If they decide to have the baby, they must decide either to raise the child or place the child for adoption. If they abort the child, they cut short an innocent life; they also expose themselves to emotional risks, and the girl to physical ones. Couples who refrain from sex do not bear those burdens and are much freer to enjoy their relationships and other aspects of their lives.

- **Freedom from pressure to marry prematurely.** One of the benefits of dating is that it helps us decide whom we want to marry. Pregnancy can pressure you to marry someone you don't know as well as you should—or even someone you'd rather not or should not marry. Even if you're sure you want to marry that person, a

pregnancy can make you rush into marriage before you're emotionally, psychologically, or financially ready.

- **Freedom from sexually transmitted diseases— including AIDS.** Chapter 4 contains a more thorough discussion of sexually transmitted diseases, but girls, in particular, should remember the following risks of sexual activity:
  - Girls are at a higher risk than boys of developing sexually transmitted diseases— for example, chlamydia, gonorrhea, herpes, or syphilis.
- Sexually experienced teenagers are three times more likely to be diagnosed as having pelvic inflammatory disease (or PID, an infection of the upper reproductive tract in women) than are twenty-five- to twenty-nine-year-old women.
- Sexually active girls under the age of sixteen are twice as likely to get cervical cancer as those who delay sexual activity until their later years.[2] At sixteen years of age and younger, cervical tissue in young women is in a transformation stage. Premarital sexual activity can be detrimental to their reproductive systems.
- **Freedom from the side effects of contraceptives/prophylactics.**[3]
  - **Condoms:** Some people are allergic to latex or to the spermicide used in certain condoms. Also, con-

doms sometimes break.

- **Diaphragms (with spermicide):** Some people are allergic to sperm-killing chemicals. Some women develop bladder infections. Some women may not be able to use a diaphragm because it cannot be fitted well. Diaphragms should not be used just after childbirth or by women who have had toxic shock syndrome.
- **Foams, creams, gels, or suppositories:** Some people are allergic to sperm-killing chemicals.
- **Intrauterine devices:** This method should generally not be used by women planning on pregnancy in the future. It should not be used by teens or by women with more than one sex partner. Insertion can be painful. It may cause heavier and more painful menstrual periods. It may increase the risk of pelvic infection. Pelvic infection can lead to tubal pregnancy or infertility. The uterus sometimes pushes IUDs out without the user knowing it.
- **The pill:** Some users notice spotting, missed periods, headaches, weight gain, nausea, breast tenderness, decreased sex drive, or depression. Heart attack, stroke, and blood clots are a risk, especially for users over thirty who smoke. This is not a good method for older women, especially if they smoke. It may increase the risk of liver tumors, gallbladder disease, and high blood pressure. It may slightly increase risk of cervical cancer. The mini-pill increases the risk of ectopic (tubal) pregnancy.
- **Sponges:** Some people are allergic to sperm-killing chemicals. This method should not be used just after childbirth or by women who have had toxic shock syndrome. This method may be less likely to work for women who have had a baby (perhaps because of a larger vagina).
- **Freedom from the guilt, doubt, disappointment, worry, and intensified feelings of rejection that are associated with unmarried sexual activity.**
  - **Guilt** from doing things that you know are wrong, even if you don't consciously admit it to yourself.
  - **Doubt** about the relationship you are involved in, wondering if it's really love or just sexual pleasure.
  - **Disappointment** with sexual intercourse itself. When sex takes place outside of marriage, worry, doubt, and guilt can ruin the enjoyment. It could be an awkward, embarrassing, or disappointing experience.
  - **Worry** about pregnancy or contracting an STD; worry about parents or others finding out about your sexual activity.
  - **Intensified rejection** when the relationship ends. Most high school relationships do end. Very few people marry their high school sweethearts. Even most college relationships end. The end of any relationship is difficult emotionally, but it hurts even more when a couple has been intimate sexually.
- **Freedom to focus your energy on establishing and accomplishing your goals.** When you are free from the physical and emotional pressures that premarital sex can bring, you will be better able to pursue any long-range plans you have for going to college or graduate school, starting a profession,

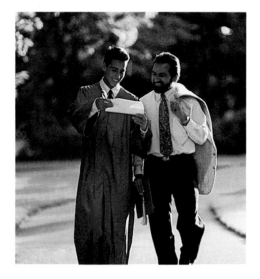

or getting married and having children.

- **Freedom to enjoy being a teenager.** The teenage years can be a great time in life. Waiting until marriage for sex will actually help you to enjoy them more.
- **Freedom to develop a better understanding of friends and to enjoy dating relationships.** In relationships involving premarital sex, many couples spend a great deal of time focusing on sex. Much of their time together may be spent in sexual activity or in discussions about it. Much of their time apart may be taken up with worry, guilt, anxiety, and regret. Freedom from these gives you the opportunity to engage in a wider range of activities and gain a broader understanding of your partner's feelings, goals, and interests. You will also have a greater opportunity to learn more about yourself.

As the above list shows, absti-

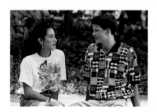

nence before marriage is physically and emotionally healthy. Far from being a sign of neurosis, abstinence dramatically increases your chance for sexual happiness later on.

Early sexual experience, on the other hand, can spell serious trouble and is often accompanied by other problems. These include alcohol and drug abuse, addiction to pornography, failing in school, and delinquency. Fortunately, however, even if you've already had premarital sex, the above benefits are not out of reach. By practicing the skills we'll cover later in this book, you can recover your sexual self-control and enjoy the freedoms associated with premarital sexual abstinence.

BREACHES OF CHARACTER

Good character, shown in sexual abstinence before marriage, can make a real difference in the quality of your life—both now and in the future. Not surprisingly, the benefits of good character are often most obvious when good character is missing. That is certainly the case with several of the behaviors listed below, behaviors that are often found in premarital sexual relationships.

MANIPULATION

How many times had Jennifer heard the words, "If you really loved me, you'd do it with me"? Too many to count, and she had always dismissed them. But this time it was different, she thought.

Jennifer, a high school senior, and Randy, also a senior, had been dating for a year. She was president of the honor society, and he was captain of the tennis

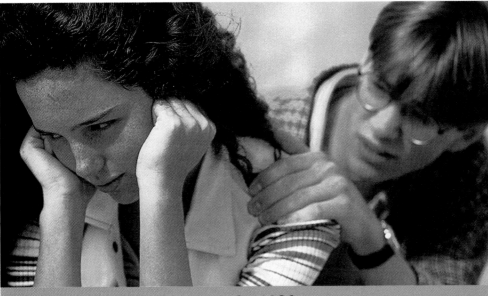

Why Say NO?

There are lots of reasons for saying NO to sex outside of marriage. Here are forty-two reasons young people have offered[4]:

1. To avoid pregnancy.
2. I'd rather say no to my boyfriend than "Yes, I'm pregnant" to my parents.
3. To avoid STDs.
4. I don't want to feel guilty.
5. I don't want the reputation of being someone that people date because they expect to have sex.
6. I would disappoint my parents.
7. I might lose respect for the other person, he or she might lose respect for me, and I might lose respect for myself.
8. Sex is better in a secure, loving marriage relationship.
9. The thought of having an abortion scares me to death.
10. Sex gets in the way of real intimate communication.
11. Sexual relationships are a lot harder to break up even when you know you should.
12. I'm afraid it may ruin a good relationship rather than make it better.
13. There are better ways to get someone to like you.
14. You won't have to worry about birth control side effects.
15. I'm not emotionally ready for that intense of a relationship.

16. I could become scared of my partner.
17. I don't want to hurt someone I really care about.
18. Sex could become the central focus of the relationship, like an addiction. At that point it is no longer a meaningful relationship, but we are using each other to satisfy sexual desires.
19. You begin to compare sexual experiences, leading to lots of disappointments.
20. I don't want to make myself vulnerable to being used or abused sexually.
21. If I'm hurt too many times, I might miss out on something great because I'm so afraid of being hurt again.
22. I like my freedom too much. Sexual relationships are binding.
23. I'm only sixteen.
24. I'm proud of my virginity, and I want to stay that way.
25. Building a relationship in other ways is more important.
26. I don't want to risk becoming someone's sex object.
27. I want my first experience to be a good one with someone who won't laugh at me, reject me, or tell lies about me, and who I know will always be there tomorrow.
28. It's possible to enjoy ourselves without getting sexually intimate.
29. Why rush into something that could be lousy or mediocre now, when it could be great later?
30. I don't want sex to lose meaning and value so that I feel "sexually bankrupt."
31. I am afraid that at this age it might not meet my expectations, and I will be seriously disappointed.
32. I don't want to risk ending a relationship by our hating each other because of it.
33. I might find it painful and the other person rough and uncaring.
34. I don't want the boy to brag about scoring with me.
35. It's the safest way not to become pregnant.
36. You may feel invaded, and you can't take it back after it's happened.
37. You may have to grow up too fast and too soon.
38. Sex may become the only thing that keeps the relationship together.
39. You may have sex too early to really enjoy or understand it.
40. You lose the chance to experience the "first time" with someone who really cares for you.
41. I want my most intimate physical relationship to be with the one I marry.
42. Sex brings feelings of jealousy, envy, and possessiveness. Every relationship changes.

team. Both teens came from respected families in the community. They shared common goals for their futures and seemed to share common values. They planned to marry after college. Jennifer said she wanted to wait until marriage to have sex, and Randy said he did too.

Following their senior prom, Jennifer and Randy attended an all-night party at the home of a classmate whose parents were out of town. Most of the other couples at the party had disappeared upstairs or out into the woods surrounding the home. Jennifer and Randy were alone in the family room watching a movie.

Normally the couple would stop kissing after a few times. But this time they didn't. In a few minutes both teens had overstepped their limits; hormones and emotions were controlling their behavior.

"Jen, come on," Randy whispered. "I know we said we'd wait, but we've gone this far. Just this once. You know I love you."

Jennifer chose to believe him.

"It was awful," she admitted months later. "It wasn't what I was expecting at all. But worse than that, I hated myself for giving in—and Randy, for talking me into something that made me feel so awful. He said it would be 'just this once.' Maybe he believed that then. But, after that first night, he expected sex every time we were alone. Our whole relationship began to revolve around sex. If I didn't want to, he would get mad, and we would argue.

"Before that night, I really loved Randy," Jennifer said, "and I thought he loved me too—partly because he had never pushed me to have sex. I thought he wanted to wait. It's not all his fault, though. I chose to give in to him, and now I've lost him. I don't care about school or even going to college. We don't see each other anymore, and I feel cheap."

This story illustrates one of the common breaches of character in sexual relations: manipulation. Both Jennifer and Randy knew the right thing to do.

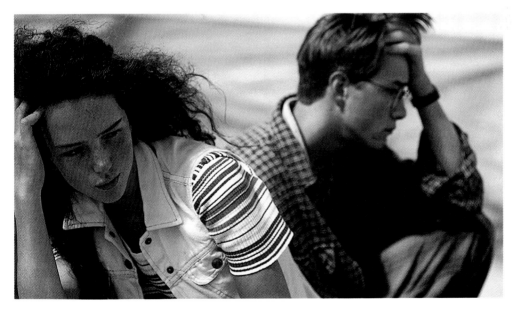

But they let their emotions get out of hand. Then Randy gave in to his passions and led Jennifer down the same path. Having done that, he continued pressuring her to have sex—to go against what he knew to be her values.

Once people let their emotions take over, it's that much easier to manipulate their partners rather than thinking of what is best for them. Instead of doing what he knew was right, Randy became selfish and manipulated his girlfriend into having sex with him by saying:

- *Just this once.* Randy may have thought it would happen only once. But, clearly, the reason he said it was to get Jennifer to have sex with him. After that night he expected to go to bed with her every time they were alone. From then on, their relationship centered on sex. When Jennifer didn't feel like it, they argued.
- *You know I love you.* Before that night, Jennifer thought she loved Randy and that he loved her— in part because he had respected her desire to save sex for marriage. But having sex proved to her that he did not love her as much as she thought. He was more interested in satisfying his desire for sexual pleasure than he was in respecting her desire to save sex for marriage.

Other statements peo-

ple use to manipulate each other into sexual relationships include:

- *Everybody's doing it.* Statements like this are intended to convince you that what the other person wants to do is actually OK or to make you feel ashamed because you're different. But the truth is, everybody is *not* doing it. In fact, some of those who say they are, really aren't. Even if everybody were doing it, however, that's no reason for you to do it.
- *You have such beautiful eyes.* Recognize the difference between a genuine compliment and flattery. A genuine compliment is meant to express sincere appreciation. Flattery is meant to influence your actions. The above line has met with success more than almost any other.
- *If you get pregnant, I'll marry you.*

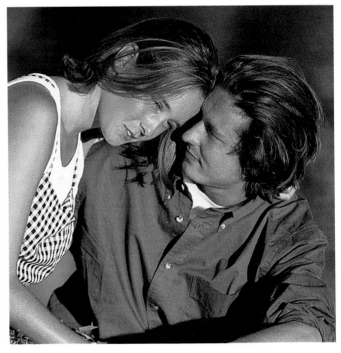

The purpose of this line is to reassure you so that you will be more willing to have sex. In the first story of this chapter, although Bryan Nikolaj didn't say those exact words to Tanya Fontaine, that was what she believed would happen. Many girls believe this line and end up with a fatherless child. The clearest answer is, "I don't want to get pregnant, and I'm not ready to get married."

- *If you won't have sex with me, I'll find someone who will.* This is a threat, plain and simple. It's easy to understand that you may not want to lose your boyfriend or girlfriend—even when he or she uses a line like this one. But everyone is worth waiting for—including you.

Boys manipulate girls, and girls manipulate boys. Anyone who tries to pressure or manipulate you into having sex is not expressing true love—or good character.

LINES AND COMEBACKS

Girl: All the boys do it. What's wrong with you?

Boy: Have you done it with all the boys? Maybe all the boys you know do it, but I don't and I'm happy with my decision.

Boy: If you really loved me, you would.

Girl: If you really loved me, you wouldn't try to manipulate me into having sex with you.

Girl: What's the matter—aren't you a man yet?

Boy: Anyone can have sex. I'm man enough to make the right decision about sex.

Boy: I'll stop when you say "stop."

Girl: "Stop!"

Boy: I won't get you pregnant.

Girl: The only way you can guarantee that is if we don't have sex. Easy enough for you to say—after all, you can't get pregnant.

Boy: We'll have safe sex.

Girl: There's no such thing. All sex is risky. I'm practicing saved sex—risk prevention, not simply risk reduction.

Boy: Why are you so worried? I'll use protection.

Girl: A condom offers about as much protection as an umbrella in a tornado. And even if it protected me from getting pregnant or sick, it wouldn't protect my heart.

Girl: It will bring us closer.

Boy: Sure, our bodies would be closer; but sex tends to break up most relationships, and I don't want to lose you.

Boy: It will only take a minute.

Girl: If you want a minute of gratification, get a microwave and cook something that tastes good.

DECEPTION OR LYING

Another breach of character in sexual relations is *deception* or *lying*. Many people who are sexually active will lie to get sex. Just as some girls will manipulate boys into having a relationship with them by giving them sex, some boys will pretend to love a girl to get sex. Even in the early stages of a relationship, a boy may tell a girl he loves her so she will feel that it's OK to have sex with him.

Besides the phrase *I love you*, other frequent lies include:
- *I'm not seeing anyone else.*
- *I've never had sex with anyone else.*
- *I've never had a sexually transmitted disease*, or *I don't have a sexually transmitted disease*, or *I just tested negative for HIV.* (Some people who know they are infected with a sexually transmitted disease do not tell a potential sex partner because they do not want to be turned down—as they rightly should be. Their sexual enjoyment is more important to them than the other person's health.)
- *I can't get pregnant now because I'm having my period*, or *I can't get pregnant now because it's right before (or after) my period.*

SELF-DECEPTION AND DENIAL

Just as we can deceive other people, so we can also deceive ourselves. Both are breaches of character. As we saw,

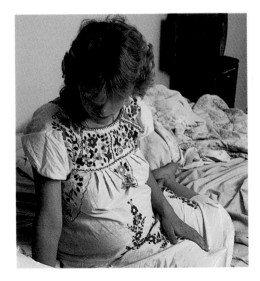

Tanya fell into *self-deception* when she talked herself into believing that Bryan would marry her once the baby was born. She denied that he was irresponsible, even though he never stayed at a job for more than a few days. Only after months of frustration at his refusal to take responsibility for their child did Tanya finally ask him to leave.

Tanya's experience is a common one. According to Child Trends, a research organization in Washington, D.C., more than 50 percent of teenage mothers are not living with the father of their child by the time the child enters elementary school, and more than 25 percent never did.[5]

The Alan Guttmacher Institute reports that in 1987 only a third of the women under the age of thirty who were raising children without their fathers received any child support.[6] Another more current study reports that only 20 percent of unwed mothers are given child support.[7]

When we talk ourselves into believing things that aren't so, we set ourselves up for serious disappointments. It's important to speak the truth to others, but it's just as important to speak the truth to ourselves. Are you telling yourself the truth when you say,

- My *partner really loves me.*
- *I won't get pregnant.*
- *I won't get an STD.*
- My *partner will stop dating other people.*
- *He'll break up with his girlfriend.*

Good character requires that we be honest with ourselves.

PORNOGRAPHY—GIGO

The rule garbage-in-garbage-out (GIGO) applies not just to computers but also to us. If we fill our minds with garbage, soon our minds won't have room for anything else. Pornography is garbage. Not only does it encourage unhealthy sexual activity and attitudes, but it also plants in our minds disturbing images that can be hard to shake—even if we want to shake them.

Young men are particularly vulnerable here. Men are much more easily "turned on" by sexually explicit images than women. That's why most pornography is directed at them. Such images can quickly trigger the release of hormones, producing powerful feelings of arousal.

Pornography is especially damaging to young men. At just the time when they need to be developing self-control, pornography arouses their sexual desire and encourages them to give in to it—regardless of who might get hurt. In addition, it encourages them to look at women as sex objects instead of as persons to be respected, loved, and cherished.

Pornography can be addictive. People who get hooked and can't stay away from it are often tempted to act out the images they've seen. This can lead to wrong and perverted sexual behavior, and even the abuse of others.

According to one ninth-grade teacher, a fourteen-year-old student sexually abused his three-year-old cousin after watching pornographic movies at home for several months. Similarly, a wife reports that her husband, even though he was well respected in the community, sexually abused their two-year-old daughter after becoming addicted to porn videos.

Pornography can also lead to sexual problems within marriage. It's hard for a wife to compete with the air-brushed, perfectly tanned, breast-implanted bodies that appear in centerfolds. As a result, men addicted to pornography can become dissatisfied with their wives and fantasize about glamorous but unreal images. Some men cannot even have sex with their wives unless they are also looking at a pornographic image. This can cause severe emotional damage to both the husband and the wife.

Because our culture is so used to pornography, people often don't see its use as a serious breach of character. But it is. By exposing ourselves to it, we are asking to be deceived, seduced, and

betrayed. It is highly deceptive. Pornographers take our sexual drives, which are normal, and redirect them in ways that are not normal. Pornography presents a twisted view of human sexuality. To expose ourselves to it willingly is a breach of character.

Pornography is bad news. It provides at best a momentary thrill, but in the end it destroys people and relationships. Pornography is garbage. If you've been filling your mind with garbage, there's only one thing to do—stop and take out the trash.[8]

PORNOGRAPHY

Pornography encourages unhealthy sexual activity and attitudes. It presents sexually explicit images and behaviors—as in a photograph or video—to arouse sexual excitement. Pornography appears in all major media of our culture, including movies, television, videos, magazines, books, computer games, and the Internet. Dolf Zillman of Indiana University and Jennings Bryant of the University of Houston have investigated the effects of pornography. They found that people who expose themselves to it are more likely to believe that:

- Sexual happiness requires no enduring commitment.
- Marriage is not a lasting and viable institution; spouses are expected to be unfaithful.
- Sex outside marriage is natural and acceptable.[9]

These beliefs and attitudes set a trap that, over time, can become highly destructive in the lives of pornography users and their family members.

DUMPING

A college student recalled his sexual experience in high school:

I finally got a girl into bed—actually it was in a car—when I was seventeen. I thought it was the hottest thing there was, but then she started saying she loved me and got clingy.

I figured out that there had probably been a dozen guys before me who thought

they had "conquered" her but who were really just objects of her need for security. That realization took all the wind out of my sails. I couldn't respect someone who gave in as easily as she did.

I was amazed to find that after four weeks of having sex as often as I wanted, I was tired of her. I didn't see any point in continuing the relationship. I finally dumped her, which made me feel even

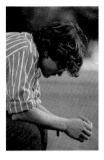

worse, because I could see that she was hurting. I felt pretty low.[10]

This story illustrates another breach of character: *dumping.* Although breaking up is often legitimate, and sometimes is a very wise move, people are not merely objects that can be discarded at will. When we begin and end our relationships for the wrong reasons, we show a profound lack of respect and compassion for the other person.

Here is what one girl wrote to "Dear Abby":

I went steady for seven months with a boy I thought was the most wonderful person in the whole world. I thought I'd always stay decent. After a while we weren't satisfied with just kissing.

He asked me to prove my love. I thought as long as we planned to be married in a few years, what would it matter?

I gave in to him, Abby, and I found out it mattered a lot. He lost all respect for me. He started going out with other girls. He even talked about me to the other boys.

Please print this for all girls to see. Maybe it will help someone who is tempted to prove her love like I did.[11]

The letter was signed "Sorry now." She put her finger on one of the main reasons a boy will leave a girl after she has given in to his demands: *He lost all respect for me.*

Actually, it's hard to imagine that he respected her in the first place. If he had really respected her, he would never have asked her to prove her love by sleeping with him.

Another reason a boy will abandon a girl after she has given in to him is the loss of a challenge—as the above college student's experience illustrated. For some, the thrill is in the chase. Once they've conquered the prize, they move on to the next challenge.

That kind of behavior reached an extreme several years ago with the Spur Posse, a gang at Lakewood High School in Southern California. Members of the gang had a running competition to see

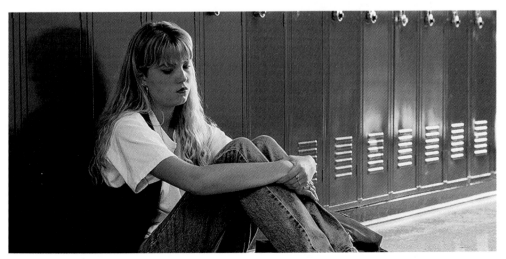

who could go to bed with the most girls. Altogether, gang members exploited hundreds of girls, some as young as ten years old. Although most of us understand that it's wrong to treat others as objects to be used and thrown away, the gang members couldn't understand why everyone was so upset when their deeds came to light. Obviously, they lacked even the most basic elements of moral knowing and moral feeling.

Again, breaking off a relationship is not necessarily bad, and sometimes it can even be a good idea. But using people as objects and simply discarding them is never right.

Part of what makes dumping so devastating is the level of commitment that sex implies. Sex can mislead a girl or a boy into thinking that the relationship is more serious than it is—that both partners truly love each other. What's more, it can create a strong emotional bond between them. When the bond is broken, deep emotional hurts remain—especially when one partner realizes that the other partner was not sincerely committed.

Young people, especially girls, often face this dilemma of being dumped: "My boyfriend is trying to get me to have sex with him. I know I shouldn't, but I don't want to lose him."

Only after it's too late does she find out that her feelings of love for him and giving herself to him won't make him love her in return. She may *think* that the best way to keep her boyfriend is to let him have his way, but she learns the hard way that it doesn't work.

Girls can also pressure boys into having sex. This was the case with Christine. Christine had never had a father who loved her or cared about her. To fill the emptiness in her heart, she sought the attention of young men. By the time she was fifteen, she had had sex with several boys. Most of the boys pretended to like her, and she settled for their short-term affection.

In her new world of sexual excitement, Christine used her body to get whatever or whomever she wanted. She thought it was a great game and enjoyed teasing and seducing the boys, especially younger ones. Sex was recreational for Christine. And several

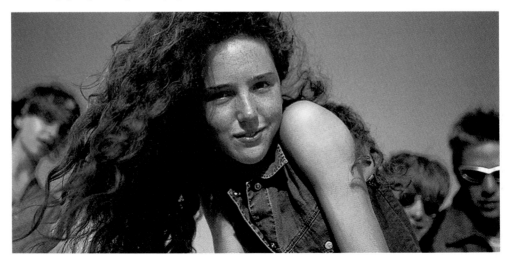

guys got burned along the way.

Christine's case is not rare. Some mothers report that their sons receive notes from girls who offer themselves to the boys. Just as surely as girls pressure boys into having sex, they also dump them.

INFIDELITY

Infidelity is another breach of character in sexual relations. It occurs when one partner in a sexual relationship has sex outside the relationship.

The story of Marcy, a fifteen-year-old girl, points out how serious infidelity can be. In a small Northern town not long ago Marcy was tried for murder. She was charged with shooting a boy in her high school.

The year before, when Marcy was a ninth grader, she dated Jud, a high school senior, the star quarterback, and one of the most popular boys at her school. Before long they started having sex. Then she heard that Jud was also having sex with other girls.

Marcy became jealous and asked Jud if the rumors were true. He laughed. This enraged her, and several days later she carried a gun to school and shot him.[12]

A similar incident took place in another town, where twenty-seven-year-old Scott faced murder charges for killing a man.

Scott and his girlfriend Trish had been living together for over a year. It was the first time Scott had been involved in a serious relationship. They planned to get married and had even made a deposit on a wedding dress.

Then one day, without warning Scott or leaving an explanation, Trish packed all of her things and moved out of their apartment.

"I was confused," he said later. "I didn't know what to do, where to turn. I couldn't eat or sleep. I made excuses not to go to work because I couldn't hold my composure."

He soon discovered that Trish was seeing another man. In a jealous rage, Scott confronted the other man and stabbed him to death.[13]

Although Marcy and Scott bear the guilt for their crimes, their partners' infidelity was a major factor. Moreover, because sex was involved in the relationships, the sense of being betrayed was much greater than if it had not been present.

COERCION

Another breach of character is *coercion*. This includes both physical force and other forms of pressure. Coercion is essentially an abuse of power.

Rape, in the legal sense of the term, is an extreme form of coercion. It is forcing sexual intercourse on a person who does not want it. Rape is punishable in nearly all societies by long-term imprisonment or death.

Rape violates the victim in a profound way. It can cause victims to suffer lifelong consequences. When someone is raped by an acquaintance, the consequences can be even more severe because the person's trust has been betrayed. Also, the victim may see the rapist in everyday, social situations.

Here is what Trish reported:

I was twenty-four years old. I knew him from college, and he was very attractive to me. We spent a lot of time together. At first we were just friends. We used to talk about each other's dating partners. We would hang out together and often go to dances or parties on the weekends. Sometimes we would kiss each other, but

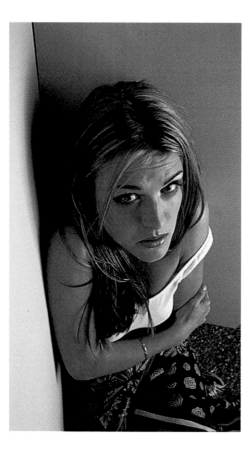

down to the floor. I laughed, too, but it was out of fear. I told him this wasn't right. He wasn't taking me seriously. I told him to stop, not once, but it seemed like a hundred times. I couldn't pull him off. After he was finished with me, he rolled over and laid on the floor. I got up crying, pulled myself together, and asked him to drive me home. On the way home I realized that I was being driven back to my house by someone who just raped me. I felt disgusted and ashamed.

I never told anyone the story. I thought everyone would blame me for what happened. I wish I could erase that night from my mind.

Victims of rape often think that their family and friends blame them. Indeed, after being raped, victims may actually question their own character. When a person has been violated by someone who was considered trustworthy, it is even more difficult to recover from the emotional wounds and feel safe or trust people again.

Our society is losing vital moral knowledge and feeling in this area. A Rhode Island survey found that among seventeen hundred middle-school children 65 percent of the boys and 49 percent of the girls stated that it was "acceptable for a man to force sex on a woman" if the couple had dated for at least six months.[14]

Many young adults have even lower standards than these children. One young man revealed his method of forcing sex on his dates. "When I pick up a girl, I drive out to a very remote place and park. Then I say, 'You've got it, and I want it. Either give it to me, or get out and start walking.'"[15]

Young people should take every precaution to ensure that they don't

nothing very serious happened. I really liked him and wished he would consider me as more than a friend, but he didn't. I could tell we were just friends because he would always want my advice about how to handle his relationship problems.

One evening we were at a party and had been drinking a lot. We decided to leave the party and watch TV in his apartment. I can remember being in the kitchen. I was getting something to eat. He came in and started joking with me. He grabbed me, and we started kissing one another. After a minute I could tell I was in trouble. He was out of control. His hands were all over my body.

He began to laugh as he pulled me

become another rape statistic. The accompanying sidebar, "Out of Harm's Way: Avoiding Acquaintance Rape," offers several such precautions.

If you are raped or someone attempts to rape you, you should get to a safe place at once and call 911 or the police. Call your parents and go to a hospital emergency room for an immediate checkup. It may take courage to report it, but you could save someone else from being raped. It's also important to get some kind of counseling from a qualified person who has experience in helping rape victims. Ask someone you trust—such as your parents, a school counselor, or someone at your church—for a recommendation.

OUT OF HARM'S WAY: AVOIDING ACQUAINTANCE RAPE

You can avoid acquaintance rape in many cases. Boys, you can avoid committing this serious offense by:
- keeping yourself away from tempting situations (see chapter 7);
- refusing to build up expectations that sexual intercourse will be part of your date;
- not assuming that your date's dress or behavior is an invitation for sex; and
- being aware of any dangerous emotions before they get out of hand.

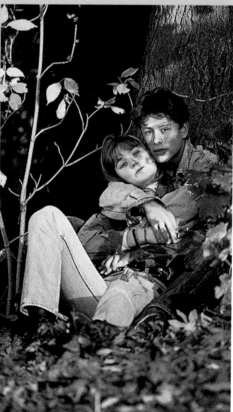

Girls, you can guard yourself against being raped by taking the following measures:

- **Avoid situations that put you at risk.**
 Avoid being in unsupervised homes. Avoid being alone in isolated places on a date. Being alone may embolden your date to force you into sex and make it harder for you to stop him.
 Don't go places where people are using alcohol or drugs—and don't use them yourself. Alcohol and drugs increase a person's desire for pleasure but decrease one's ability to make good, rational decisions. One study shows that 75 percent of the men and 55 percent of the women involved in date rape had been drinking and/or taking drugs before the incident.[16]

- **Become safety conscious.**

Be sure to lock your car when you get out and check it carefully before getting in. Park close to building entrances and away from vans or other vehicles where predators can easily conceal themselves.

Stay in well-lighted areas at night. Avoid going to dark, "romantic" places and parking—that spells danger! If possible, be with friends, not alone. Let your parents know where you're going, when you'll be home, and whom you'll be with.

- **Avoid actions that are sexually stimulating.**

A person can misinterpret certain kinds of physical touching. Someone may assume you want to engage in sexual intercourse when you intend only to communicate friendship.

How you dress and how you act can be misinterpreted also. Dress with respect—for yourself and for your date. Your clothing may unintentionally arouse your date. Both women and men should be cautious about how they dress and act when they're on a date, or in any situation. Avoid sending mixed signals. Clothing does talk, whether you intend it to or not.

Keep in mind that some men and women may find it hard to distinguish between casual friendliness and a sexual invitation. Men are more likely to assume that friendliness implies sexual attraction.

- **Avoid teasing.**

Try not to get a person's attention by teasing. Teasing can easily be misinterpreted. It may focus the other person's attention on the physical.

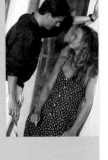

- **Listen to your gut feelings.**

Acquaintance rape victims report having had a strange feeling about the person, the situation, or some other circumstance, but they did not pay attention to the feeling. Be willing to listen to that feeling.

- **Be aware of the physiological and psychological differences whereby men and women are aroused.**

Teen boys often have a stronger desire than girls for physical touch, as well as stronger and more immediate sexual feelings.[17] Young men usually reach the peak of their sexual desire between the ages of seventeen and nineteen. Young women reach their peak at twenty-eight years or older. Girls tend to want more signs of affection, such as holding hands or hugging. Girls usually consider sexual relationships to be more serious than boys do.[18]

Young people do not always understand how differences between the sexes are expressed in relationships. Boys tend to be more visual and are thus more easily aroused by what they see. That's why it's important for girls to dress appropriately. But no matter how a girl dresses, there's no excuse for forcing sex upon her.

- **Be able to identify manipulative or coercive statements:**
  "If you won't have sex, then I'll find someone who really loves me."
  "I thought you said you loved me."
  "I have protection; don't be scared."
  "Why are you being a tease?"
  Such statements are manipulative and self-serving; they put the other person on the defensive. No one who has your best interest in mind will pressure you with statements like these.

- **Say no to sexual pressure and mean it.**
  Be assertive. Communicate your feelings loudly and clearly. Use consistent body language and a strong tone of voice. No means *no* in what you say and what you do. It does not mean *yes* or *maybe*. Be straightforward and consistent in saying *no*. Your date may not like hearing you say *no* and may feel frustrated. But a true friend will understand. If a person won't take *no* for an answer, you are better off without that person.

VIOLATING ONE'S OWN OR ANOTHER'S CONSCIENCE

A common thread in most of the character breaches described in this chapter is one person trying to get another to do something that violates his or her conscience. In fact, *the whole point of using manipulation, lying, deception, or coercion is to overcome someone else's scruples about having sex.* When that person succeeds, he or she does so at the cost of the other person's conscience. Even in cases of rape, when victims have done nothing to violate their conscience, many of them nonetheless *feel* as if they have.

When we engage in the behaviors described in this chapter, we also violate our conscience. This is clear from many of the preceding stories. Jennifer had decided to wait until she and Randy were married before engaging in sexual intercourse. She felt "awful" and "cheap" when she gave in to Randy's pressure. The girl in the Dear Abby letter said she had expected to "stay decent." She found that having sex without being married "mattered a lot." The college student "felt pretty low" when he saw how much he had hurt the girl he dumped after getting tired of having sex with her. Clearly, violating your own conscience and causing others to violate theirs is the opposite of love and respect.

In this chapter we have seen that sexuality can't be separated from character. In the next three chapters we will look more closely at some of the ways your own character in the area of sexuality can affect you now and in the future.

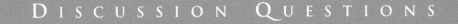

DISCUSSION QUESTIONS

1. There's a saying: "If you stick your hand in the cookie jar, you'll eventually end up taking the cookie." If you want to avoid premarital sex, you need to avoid situations where you're more likely to give in to sex. What are such situations? How can you avoid them?

2. When a woman says she "won't go all the way," or a man says he'll "only go as far as you want," are they saying NO to sex or MAYBE? How do you tell the difference between NO and MAYBE?

3. Why do people often feel "cheap," "awful," and "depressed" after engaging in premarital sex? Is guilt healthy?

4. Premarital sex can lead to sexual problems later within marriage, including guilt, shame, and disappointment. Why do you think this happens?

5. Is sex worth waiting for in a loving, committed, and monogamous relationship, traditionally known as marriage? Discuss your answer.

6. How does avoiding premarital sex safeguard your ability to have children?

CHAPTER

I believe that having sex before marriage is too dangerous and risky...
If I could make everyone's decision for them, I would choose for
everyone to wait. I can't make everyone's decision, but I have made
mine. I have chosen not to have sex because I feel that there are too many
negative consequences, and I also feel I am not emotionally ready for it.

RISKY BUSINESS: SEXUALLY

-A high school senior, West Springfield, Virginia

TRANSMITTED DISEASES

Most people do not set out to destroy the physical and emotional well-being of themselves and others. But when you have sex outside of marriage, you are risking your health *and* the health of the other person.

In the previous chapter we discussed several breaches of character. In this chapter and the next two we'll look at another breach of character: *putting yourself or another person at risk.* Being aware of the facts as well as the possible consequences of your actions is part of moral knowing. And not wanting to put yourself or another person at risk is part of moral feeling.

Risk-taking in sexual behavior has both physical and emotional consequences. The physical consequences fall into two broad types: sexually transmitted disease and pregnancy. In this chapter we will focus on sexually transmitted disease and condoms. In chapter 5 we will focus on pregnancy and its aftermath.

SEXUALLY TRANSMITTED DISEASE IN THE UNITED STATES

In the last thirty years, sexually transmitted disease (STD) has become epidemic. Back in the 1960s syphilis and

gonorrhea, both treatable with penicillin, were the most prevalent STDs. Today more than twenty STDs are widespread throughout the United States. Twelve million people in the United States are newly infected with a sexually transmitted disease every year.[1] Three million, or about one-fourth, of those new infections occur among teenagers. This means that about 25 percent of sexually active teens—or about 13 percent of all teens—are newly infected each year.[2] As a sexually active teen you're more likely to contract an STD than you are to kill yourself playing Russian roulette with a six-shooter.

When statistics include everyone under the age of twenty-five, the number of newly infected people jumps to roughly eight million a year, which is about two-thirds of all new infections.

Tragically, about a million people in the United States are currently infected with the human immunodeficiency virus (HIV), the virus that causes AIDS.[3] No less tragic, about fifty-six million people in the United States are

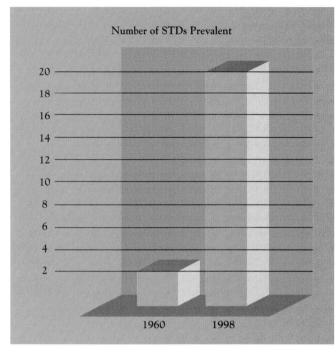

Number of STDs Prevalent

20
18
16
14
12
10
8
6
4
2

1960   1998

PID also increases a woman's chance of having a tubal/ectopic pregnancy. What happens is this. Through scarring from PID, a fertilized egg gets "snagged" in the fallopian tube. Instead of implanting itself in the woman's uterus, the embryo begins to grow in the tube. This is a life-threatening condition. Symptoms include severe lower abdominal pain and vaginal spotting. If left untreated, the growing fetus will eventually rupture the tube, causing severe internal bleeding and requiring emergency surgery. According to the National Institute of Allergy and Infectious Diseases (NIAID), a large proportion of the 70,000 tubal pregnancies that occur every year are caused by PID.[6]

Each year PID and its complications affect from 750,000 to a million women.[7] Teenage girls bear the brunt of this epidemic. A sexually active fifteen-year-old girl is about ten times as likely to develop pelvic inflammatory disease as a twenty-four-year-old.[8]

currently infected with a sexually transmitted virus *other than* HIV. That's about one in every five people you see on the street. Diseases caused by bacteria—such as chlamydia, gonorrhea, and syphilis—also exist in distressingly high numbers.

Among women a frequent consequence of some STDs is pelvic inflammatory disease (PID), an infection of the upper reproductive tract. It occurs when certain germs, including those that cause chlamydia and gonorrhea, spread upward through the genital tract—from the vagina or cervix through the uterus to the fallopian tubes, and even into nearby organs, including the appendix, liver, and spleen.[4] A single episode of PID carries a 25 percent chance of infertility; a second infection carries a 50 percent chance; and a third infection carries a 75 percent chance, according to a report from the Medical Institute for Sexual Health.[5]

Why are STDs so much more prevalent today than thirty years ago? Mainly because more people are having sex outside of marriage, and they're having it with more partners. As the former surgeon general of the United States C. Everett Koop emphasized, sexual activity outside a monogamous relationship is risky because every time a person has sex with a partner, that person is having sex with everyone the partner

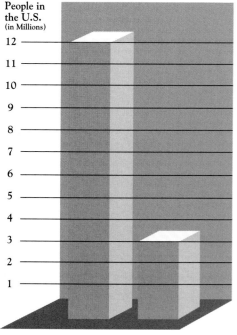

People in the U.S.
(in Millions)

12
11
10
9
8
7
6
5
4
3
2
1

People newly infected with STDs every year

Teens newly infected with STDs every year

has had sex with.[9]

Another reason for the increase is that the majority of people who are infected have no obvious symptoms, so they don't know they are contagious.[10] And many of those who do know they're infected don't tell—as we saw in chapter 3 when we discussed deception and lying.

In addition to the growing number of people with STDs, many STDs that were once uncommon have now become widespread. Most people, of course, know about HIV/AIDS. But there are many other sexually transmitted diseases. These diseases may also have serious physical consequences, including sterility, birth defects, cancer, and death. Some of them have no known cure.

What follows is a discussion of some of the more common STDs. For a brief summary of important facts about STDs, see the sidebar "STD Facts in Brief."

STD FACTS IN BRIEF

Here are some quick facts on sexually transmitted diseases, including the number of new cases reported each year and some of the consequences for the infected individual.[11]

NONVIRAL CURABLE DISEASES

Chlamydia
New cases per year: About 4,000,000.
Consequences:
• Women may suffer PID, tubal pregnancy, chronic pelvic pain, and infertility.

- Men may experience epididymo-orchitis, an acute inflammation of a testicle and the coiled tube that carries sperm from the testicle. Epididymo-orchitis may cause sterility.
- Both men and women run a greater risk of HIV infection if exposed to the virus.
- Unborn and newborn babies may suffer premature delivery, pneumonia, and neonatal eye infections.

Trichomoniasis
New cases per year: About 3,000,000.
Consequences:
- Both men and women have an increased risk of being infected with HIV if they are exposed to the virus.
- Unborn and newborn babies may suffer premature delivery.

Gonorrhea
New cases per year: About 1,500,000.
Consequences:
- Women may suffer PID and tubal pregnancy.
- Both men and women may experience infertility and infection of their joints, heart valves, or brain. They also run a greater risk of HIV infection if they are exposed.
- Unborn and newborn babies may suffer blindness, meningitis (inflammation of the membranes that envelop the brain and the spinal cord), and septic arthritis (inflammation of joints caused by an infection).

Syphilis
New cases per year: Variable. According to the Centers for Disease Control (CDC) there were 11,624 new cases in 1996.
Consequences:
- Men and women risk serious damage to body organs, as well as mental illness, and run a greater risk of HIV infection if they are exposed.
- Unborn and newborn babies may suffer stillbirth or neonatal death, active syphilis, and damage to the heart, brain, or eyes.

Chancroid
New cases per year: About 35,000.
Consequences:
- Both men and women run a greater risk of being infected with HIV if they are exposed to the virus.
- Consequences for unborn and newborn babies are unknown.

Human papillomavirus (HPV)
New cases per year: 500,000 to 1,000,000.
Consequences:
- In women HPV can cause cancer of the cervix, vulva, vagina, or anus.
- In men HPV may cause cancer of the penis or anus.
- Unborn and newborn babies may suffer warts in the throat, which can block their air passages.

Genital herpes
New cases per year: 200,000 to 500,000.
Consequences:
- Men and women run a greater risk of HIV infection if exposed.
- Unborn and newborn babies may suffer premature delivery, serious brain damage, and death.

Hepatitis B
New cases per year: About 300,000.
Consequences:
- Men and women may experience cirrhosis, liver cancer, and immune system disorders.
- Unborn and newborn babies may suffer liver disease and liver cancer.

Human immunodeficiency virus (HIV)
New cases per year: 40,000 to 50,000.
Consequences:
- Men and women may suffer a variety of disorders, including acquired immune deficiency syndrome (AIDS), which leaves patients extremely vulnerable to various forms of cancer and to a wide range of infectious diseases.
- Unborn and newborn babies may also suffer immune system disorders and AIDS.

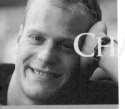
STDs and Your Future

STDs can lead to...
- pelvic inflammatory disease (PID)
- cervical cancer
- tubal/ectopic pregnancies
- sterility
- damage of major body organs
- death

If the mother is infected, babies can suffer...
- blindness
- infection
- pneumonia
- premature birth
- mental retardation
- death

NOTE: *A baby can contract an STD from the mother while in the uterus or during delivery. For those STDs which have a cure, once the mother is cured and not reinfected by another partner, the disease cannot be passed on to future children.*

Bacterial STDs

Chlamydia

Joella entered her family doctor's office. She was a high school student and had been dating one of the most popular boys at her school. Shortly after they started having sex, Joella began experiencing pain in her abdomen. Thinking it was gonorrhea, her family doctor prescribed antibiotics. But she kept having pain, so he continued to treat her for a year. Eventually, when the pain did not stop, Joella's family doctor referred her to a gynecologist.

The gynecologist was able to spot the cause of Joella's pelvic inflammatory disease. It was chlamydia, not gonorrhea as the family doctor had suspected. With the

right antibiotics her pain disappeared.

Although Joella no longer has the infection, she probably has scars on her fallopian tubes and ovaries. The scars, along with adhesions (which occur when the sides of the tubes stick together), will most likely prevent her from having children unless she goes through an expensive and troublesome fertility process.

What is chlamydia, and what are the dangers for someone infected with the disease?

Chlamydia is a name for several strains of the bacterium *Chlamydia trachomatis*. Chlamydial infections are the most common of all the sexually transmitted diseases, with about four million new cases every year.[12] The highest rate of infection occurs among teenagers. It is estimated that 10 percent of all ado-

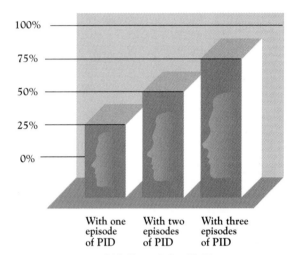

Occurrence of Infertility Among Women

100%

75%

50%

25%

0%

With one
episode
of PID

With two
episodes
of PID

With three
episodes
of PID

(Medical Institute for Sexual Health)

In men, chlamydia can lead to epididymo-orchitis, an acute inflammation of a testicle and its epididymis, the small coiled tube that carries sperm from the testicle. Epididymo-orchitis is marked by pain or tenderness and swelling of the testicle. One possible outcome of epididymo-orchitis is sterility.

In both men and women, a chlamydial infection can facilitate the transmission of HIV.

Gonorrhea

Jan noticed a burning pain when urinating and a pus-like discharge from her urethra. A culture taken by her doctor confirmed the diagnosis: gonorrhea.

Jan had engaged in sex for the first time the previous weekend. Her symptoms appeared in a few days, but they could have waited a few months to appear. Even if she displayed no symptoms, she could still transmit the disease to another sexual partner. Roughly 80 percent of men and women who have gonorrhea are unaware of its presence in the various stages.

Gonorrhea infected Jan's vulva, urethra, bladder, vagina, and cervix, causing a vaginal discharge. She was fortunate that it didn't reach her uterus, tubes, and ovaries (pelvic inflammatory disease), closing her tubes.

Jan learned later that her infected sexual partner had experienced no symptoms at first. But he, too, developed burning when urinating as well as

lescent girls—and 20 to 40 percent of sexually active teenage girls—are infected with chlamydia. This epidemic, however, is largely a silent one. As many as 75 percent of infected women and 25 percent of infected men have few or no evident symptoms.[13]

Among adults, chlamydia is spread through sexual intercourse, although children born to infected women may develop serious eye infections or pneumonia.

In women, the disease affects mainly the uterus, fallopian tubes, and ovaries, where it may lead to PID and all of its consequences, such as scarring, infertility, and the risk of tubal pregnancy. Chlamydia may also cause damage and scarring even when no symptoms of PID are present. Other complications for women include miscarriage and premature birth.

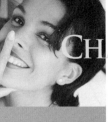

a need to urinate often. He eventually had a heavy, pus-like secretion from the penis, a further symptom of gonorrhea.

Gonorrhea is an STD brought on by the pus-producing bacterium *gonococcus*.[14] It is one of the earliest known diseases. Hippocrates wrote about it 2,400 years ago, and descriptions of the disease survive from even earlier times. After the introduction of effective antibiotics, gonorrhea was expected to become a thing of the past. But after a period of decline, the disease is once again on the rise. Since 1965, in fact, the number of gonorrhea cases has almost doubled. The annual rate of new infections stands at about 1.5 million.[15]

Symptoms of gonorrhea vary. Many people show no symptoms at all. In men, however, symptoms usually include painful or difficult urination and a pus-filled discharge from the urethra. Scarring of the urethra may cause lingering urinary tract problems.

In women, the most common symptoms include painful or difficult urination, a pus-filled vaginal discharge, bleeding between periods, excessive menstrual bleeding, or any combination of the above. Infected women may also develop PID, the scarring from which may cause pelvic pain during menstruation and intercourse. If such pain continues, or if the gonorrhea does not respond to antibiotics, the woman may have to undergo a hysterectomy, leaving her irreversibly sterile.

Men and women who engage in anal intercourse can develop rectal infections from the disease. Symptoms include diarrhea, painful bowel movements, anal irritation, and pus in the stool. Infected men and women who have oral sex can spread the disease to

the mouth and throat. Gonorrhea can cause other complications such as rash, high fever, and arthritis, which in some cases even require hospitalization.

In pregnant women, gonorrhea may cause a miscarriage or premature delivery. At birth, the gonococcus bacterium can infect the eyes of the baby during passage through the birth canal, resulting in blindness if untreated.

In adults, the gonococcus bacterium is transmitted almost exclusively by sexual intercourse and is very contagious. A person who has sex even once with an infected partner has a 40 percent chance of being infected. Antibiotics can usually eliminate the infection, but recently the bacterium has grown increasingly resistant to them.

SYPHILIS

Amber stepped into the college clinic and glanced about nervously. She hoped no one would recognize her. After having sex with a fellow student, Amber now had a small but painless genital sore.

The clinic physician took a sample and sent it to a lab for testing. The report that came back indicated simply an inflammation. The lab, however, had failed to test for syphilis.

Since the lesion remained, the clinic doctor referred Amber to a gynecologist, who suspected syphilis. Further tests confirmed his suspicions.

In this instance, penicillin cured Amber's syphilis. Left untreated, however, the syphilis infection could have led to arthritic-like symptoms; blindness; insanity; paralysis; bone deterioration; fatal bone, blood vessel, and heart damage; and death.

The bacterium *Treponema pallidum* causes syphilis. Although the disease

STD	Symptoms Male/Female	Complications	Complications to Infected Babies†	Treatment	Prevention
SYPHILIS	Painless sores; rash and fever	Severe damage to the brain and body organs; heart disease; paralysis; insanity and death. Destructive skin, liver and lung tumors.	Deafness and crippling by bone disease. 25% will die in the uterus.	Antibiotics: Penicillin Other	Sexual self-control before and after marriage
GONORRHEA	Burning sensation during urination Males: discharge from penis Females: discharge from vagina Many people have NO symptoms.	Sterility can occur in both sexes. Males: urethral damage and joint infections. Females: ectopics, PID (pelvic inflammatory disease), death.	Blindness	Antibiotics: Penicillin Ampicillin Doxycycline Other	Sexual self-control before and after marriage
CHLAMYDIA	Pain during urination. Males: discharge from penis; inflammation of urinary tract Females: discharge from vagina Many show NO symptoms.	Males: inflammation of male organs, which can lead to sterility. Females: tubal pregnancies, PID; infertility.	Eye, ear and lung infections; pneumonia; conjunctivitis	Antibiotics: Doxycycline Other	Sexual self-control before and after marriage

† Babies can contract STDs during pregnancy or birth from the mother.

was once feared the way AIDS is today, modern antibiotics dramatically curtailed its spread after World War II. The number of new infections began increasing again in the mid-1950s, hitting a high of about 20 new infections for every 100,000 people in 1990. Since then, however, the rate of infections has plummeted to a low of 4.4 new infections per 100,000 in 1996.[16] The reason for the decline is unclear.

In adults, syphilis is passed almost exclusively through sexual contact: kissing, vaginal and anal intercourse, and oral-genital touch. But the disease may also be passed from mother to child during pregnancy, where it can cause miscarriage, stillbirth, or serious physical and mental problems after birth.

The first sign of syphilis infection is the appearance of a painless open sore, or chancre, which usually shows up near the site of the infection, such as the vulva, vagina, or penis. In men, the chancre usually appears in visible locations, making early detection relatively easy. In women, however, the chancre may appear high inside the vagina, where it usually goes unnoticed.

The chancre may appear any time from ten days to three months after exposure, although it usually appears after about three weeks. A few weeks later, it usually disappears, with or without treatment.

Weeks or months after the chancre

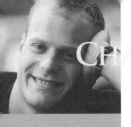

has disappeared, a range of new symptoms may occur, including low-grade fever, sore throat, fatigue, headache, swollen lymph glands, a rash on the skin or mucous membranes, a mild inflammation of the liver, and hair loss. These symptoms may come and go for up to two years. But even without treatment, they eventually disappear.

After this, some people experience no further problems. Others, however, experience serious consequences, including damage to joints, eyes, heart, and nervous system. The damage may go undetected for a long time. But once detected at this late stage in the disease, the damage is usually severe and irreversible.

Syphilis is readily cured with antibiotics if it is caught in the early stages. But, as we saw in Amber's case, early-stage syphilis can be easily misdiagnosed because its symptoms are similar to those of many other ailments. Because of this, people need to inform their doctors about any sexual activity they've had.

VIRAL STDs

HUMAN PAPILLOMAVIRUS

Eighteen-year-old Mary Ann entered the office of a gynecologist. She was referred to him after her family doctor diagnosed her with a sexually transmitted disease. She had growths on her vulva which the gynecologist determined were venereal warts caused by the human papillomavirus (HPV).

Because the doctor saw Mary Ann in the early stages of the disease, he was able to get rid of the warts by applying the chemical podophyllin. Had she waited, treatment might have taken

much longer and cost more, and the warts might have been more difficult to eliminate. Some women do not go to a doctor until the warts are extremely large.

Like Mary Ann, Carol was diagnosed early enough. When she visited her gynecologist for her annual check-up, a Pap smear found precancerous cells—caused by HPV—on her cervix. (A Pap smear is a test used to detect abnormalities in the cells of the cervix.) Early discovery and treatment prevented the precancerous cells in Carol's cervix from developing into cervical cancer, which afflicts over sixteen thousand women every year and kills about five thousand.[17]

Genital warts also afflict men. Consider the story of John, a young man who had never heard of HPV. After he and his girlfriend had sex one time, small bumps appeared on his penis. From his doctor he learned that an HPV infection caused the genital warts.

To remove the warts John spent a lot of time, experienced a lot of discomfort, and lost a lot of money on acid treatment, laser procedures, and surgery—to no avail. He still has the warts. He worries that he may develop cancer and, because of the warts, wonders if he should ever marry.[18]

Human papillomavirus is one of the most common sexually transmitted diseases. According to the National Institute of Allergy and Infectious Diseases (NIAID), as many as 40 million people in the United States are infected with HPV—that's about one in every six people you see on the street. A high percentage of sexually active people have HPV. What's more, the number of infected people appears to be rising.[19]

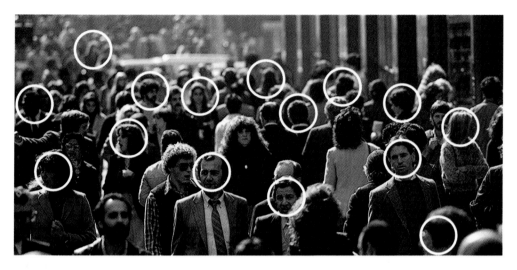

The *Journal of Adolescent Health* reported that the estimated number of private office visits for teenagers with HPV rose from fifty thousand in 1966 to three hundred thousand in 1989.[20]

A report from the Medical Institute for Sexual Health estimates that between 40 and 50 percent of sexually active teenage girls have been infected with HPV.[21] A study at the University of California at Berkeley found that fully 46 percent of female students visiting the university's gynecology clinic were infected with HPV.[22]

An HPV infection may produce soft warts on or around the genital organs. These warts are highly contagious. In men the warts may appear on the penis, the scrotum, or around the anus. In women the warts may appear on the vulva and labia, inside the vagina, on the cervix, or around the anus. Warts may also appear in the mouth and throat when there has been oral sexual contact with an infected person.[23]

HPV can cause cervical cancer. In fact, HPV is the leading risk factor for cervical cancer and accounts for 90 per-cent of all cases.[24] Genital HPV infec-tion can also lead to cancers of the vulva and vagina in women, and cancers of the penis and scrotum in men.

There is no cure for an HPV infec-tion. Although warts may be treated and removed, the virus remains.

Condoms offer little or no protection against HPV. "Outercourse," in which there is genital contact but no penetra-tion, is also unsafe. HPV is transmitted not only through sexual fluids, but also by skin-to-skin contact in the entire genital region, including the vagina, vulva, penis, scrotum, and surrounding areas.[25]

Herpes

Tina visited her doctor for a check-up and complained of painful sores on her vulva. The blisters had appeared after she received cortisone injections for another health problem. Doing a culture confirmed her doctor's suspicions: she had herpes.

Tina had probably been infected with the herpes virus during a sexual rela-tionship she had had many years earlier. In Tina's case, the cortisone injections activated the blisters. To prevent further outbreaks, Tina took acyclovir, an expensive drug, three or four times a day for a year. If she experiences more outbreaks of the painful blisters, she will have to take acyclovir again for another year.

Like HPV, the viruses that cause genital herpes, herpes simplex virus I and herpes simplex virus II are widespread.[26] NIAID puts the number of infected Americans at about thirty million. Other researchers have estimated that anywhere from 20 to 40 percent of whites and 30 to 60 percent of non-whites may be infected with type II.[27] Moreover, the rate of infection is perhaps 5 to 10 percent higher in women than in men.[28]

Infection with a herpes simplex virus (HSV) may lead to painful sores and blisters in or on the genital organs. In men, herpes blisters may affect the penis, scrotum, or anus. In women, blisters may appear on the vulva, inside the vagina, on the cervix, or in the anal area. Outbreaks may also appear in any location on the skin of men and women.

Outbreaks may be triggered by stress, illness, tight clothes, intercourse, menstruation, or other factors like the cortisone injection that activated Tina's infection. The outbreaks are usually preceded by pain, tingling, burning, or itching. Once the blisters have developed, they break open and may leave sores up to an inch wide. A woman may find that the first outbreak of herpes is so painful that she cannot urinate. She may need to be hospitalized for medication and a catheterization (a procedure in which a tube is inserted into the urethra to facilitate urination).

Herpes is spread by sexual contact with an infected partner who is *shedding*, or giving off, the virus. Shedding occurs just before and during an outbreak. It may also occur in people who have no symptoms whatever. As a result, many people are unknowingly infecting their partners.

Herpes may also be spread from mother to infant during birth. The infection occurs as the baby passes through the cervix and vagina. When herpes is spread this way, the virus may attack the nervous system of the baby, resulting in permanent brain damage or death. Any woman who is pregnant and has herpes needs to tell her doctor.

As with HPV, herpes is incurable.

HIV/AIDS

The first case of acquired immune deficiency syndrome (AIDS) in the United States was reported in 1981,[29] and in the next few years the disease exploded across the country.

By that time, Jerry was tired of his homosexual lifestyle. With the threat of AIDS he decided to make a change. But he was too late. He was already infected with the human immunodeficiency virus (HIV), the virus that causes AIDS.

Sad and shocked, Jerry told his doctor that from 1984 to 1987, after he gave up the homosexual lifestyle, he had sex with six women. In all probability he had contracted HIV during his years as a homosexual and had carried the deadly disease without knowing it. Every female sexual partner since then was in danger of being infected.

Jerry knew that three of the six women had married and two were prostitutes. He knew nothing about the sixth woman. If infected, the two prostitutes have probably infected some of their customers. Likewise, the three married women may have infected their husbands. And so on.

Networking is a fact of life with sexually transmitted diseases. When you have sex with someone, you are essentially having sex with everyone that person has had sex with, as well as with all the people *their* sexual partners have slept with. You are connected with every other person in the network. If anyone in the network was infected with HIV, then you are also in danger of getting HIV.

Once someone becomes HIV-positive—infected with the virus—that person has the disease and is contagious for life. That person can infect others through sexual contact, transfusions, broken skin, or shared drug needles.

The following stories illustrate how AIDS affected two men.

Frank lay in his bed, waiting to die. He weighed ninety-three pounds. His bones protruded from his body; his eyes sank into dark sockets. Towels soaking in sweat lay underneath him. He waited for sporadic visits from a friend who brought him money and food. He was thirty-eight. Most of his friends had successful lives, but he was close to the end. He didn't care anymore.

"I look forward to it," he said. "I wish it would happen tomorrow. I have no life."[30]

"We're all going to die," a team leader in a San Francisco hospice for AIDS patients said.

Other patients in the hospice lay in silence, smoking cigarettes and hugging teddy bears. Ed smoked about three packs of cigarettes a day. Fresh flowers and a photograph of his parents adorned his otherwise sparse room. Ed, too, was waiting to die, just like the others. His body had become so shriveled that he all but vanished among the bedcovers.[31]

A 1996 study estimates that 650,000 to 900,000 people in the United States were living with an HIV infection in 1992.[32] Since the beginning of the AIDS epidemic in the United States, over a half million cases of AIDS and 362,004 deaths in the United States have been reported to the Centers for

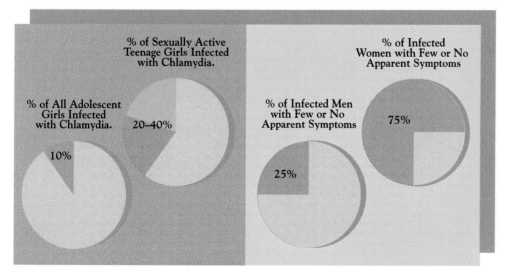

% of Sexually Active Teenage Girls Infected with Chlamydia.

% of Infected Women with Few or No Apparent Symptoms

% of All Adolescent Girls Infected with Chlamydia.

20–40%

% of Infected Men with Few or No Apparent Symptoms

75%

10%

25%

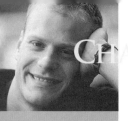

Disease Control and Prevention.[33] Approximately 50,000 of those deaths occurred in 1995 alone.

In the United States, AIDS is currently the leading cause of death among people ages twenty-five to forty-four.[34] Since it can take over ten years for an HIV infection to turn into AIDS, many of these deaths came from infections acquired by people during their teen years. In fact, 25 percent of all new HIV infections are found in people under the age of twenty-two.

Initial signs of HIV infection may include a variety of flu-like symptoms, including fever, sore throat, headaches, fatigue, nausea, diarrhea, achiness, and irritability. These symptoms may show up anywhere from a few days to three months after exposure and last about two or three weeks. Many people show no symptoms at all. And if symptoms appear, they can easily be mistaken for flu.

After the initial symptoms have passed, there may be no outward indications of infection. A person infected with HIV may feel perfectly healthy and have no idea that he or she is carrying the disease. Blood tests may indicate an HIV infection, but usually not until one to six months after a person has been exposed to the virus. Some people have gone even longer before a blood test detected anything.

This symptom-free stage may last anywhere from a few months to many years. The average time is about ten years, although some people infected in the early 1980s remain symptom-free to this day.

In most people, however, HIV gradually destroys the immune system's ability to fight off infection and cancer. AIDS occurs when the destruction reaches a point where the infected person can no longer fight off diseases that are easily repelled by people with intact immune systems.

Eventually, the infected person may show signs of HIV-symptomatic disease.[35] These symptoms include enlarged lymph nodes, fever that has no identifiable source, diarrhea, weight loss, fatigue, fungal mouth infections, and shingles (a painful condition that occurs when the virus that causes chicken pox is reactivated—usually because a person's immune system has been weakened by old age, cancer and cancer treatments, or HIV infection).

As the immune system becomes even weaker, the actual symptoms of AIDS appear. At this point the immune system is overwhelmed by germs that are normally harmless to healthy people. Some of the resulting diseases include pneumocystis pneumonia, toxoplasmosis, mycobacterium avium complex, and a variety of cytomegalovirus diseases.

AIDS sufferers are also vulnerable to several forms of cancers, including various non-Hodgkin's lymphomas (cancers of the lymph system) and Kaposi's sarcoma, which is most commonly found in homosexual men with AIDS but may be found in others as well. Cervical cancer is also found in many women with AIDS.

Fifty percent of AIDS victims die within a year after these symptoms first appear. Ninety percent die within three years. About 30 percent of the babies born to HIV-infected mothers are born with HIV. Most do not live beyond a few years. There is no cure for AIDS.

The AIDS virus is most often spread through direct sexual contact. This includes genital and anal intercourse, oral-genital contact, and open-mouth and "French" kissing (because of the possible presence of blood and sores or cuts in the mouth).

Some people maintain that oral sex is safe, but this is untrue. "There has been an unfortunate misinterpretation in some quarters that because epidemiological studies suggest it is easier to get infected by anal than oral sex, people think oral sex is in fact safe," says Anthony S. Fauci, chief of the NIAID. "That is a fundamentally wrong assumption."[36]

A 1996 study provides strong evidence that people who engage in oral sex risk being infected with the AIDS virus through the mouth, even when they have no bleeding gums or oral sores. According to Ruth M. Ruprecht, an immunologist at the Dana-Farber Cancer Institute in Boston, the study "shows conclusively that the AIDS virus can enter the body through the mouth, find its way into the bloodstream, and cause AIDS."[37]

No sex is safe when one partner has HIV.

HEPATITIS B

Hepatitis B is one of the most common sexually transmitted diseases in the world. Every year an estimated 300,000 people in the United States become infected with the hepatitis B virus (HBV).[38]

Symptoms of hepatitis B range from mild to severe. About a third of all cases are *silent*, with no evident symptoms. Early symptoms, when they occur, include headache, low-grade fever, aches,

SEXUALLY TRANSMITTED DISEASES — VIRAL

STD	Symptoms Male/Female	Complications	Complications to Infected Babies†	Treatment	Prevention
HPV Venereal Warts	White or gray warts appearing on the penis, cervix, vagina and vulva Many people show NO symptoms.	Cancer of the cervix, vulva, penis, vagina and anus. Warts may reappear for a lifetime.	Warts on the larynx	There is no cure. The warts can be removed by podophyllin, trichloracetic acid or laser.	Sexual self-control before and after marriage
GENITAL HERPES	Both males and females: blisters and sores, fever, headaches, pain while urinating. Females: vaginal discharge, painless sores on the cervix.	Sores may appear for a lifetime.	Blindness, brain damage, nerve damage	Oral acyclovir helps healing. No cure.	Sexual self-control before and after marriage
HEPATITIS B	Headache, fever, nausea. Later symptoms: abdominal pain, yellowing of eyes.	Cancer of the liver	Pass disease on to baby	Vaccine	Sexual self-control before and after marriage
AIDS	Weight loss, fever, tiredness, swollen glands and diarrhea.	Destroys immune system. Death usually caused by cancer or infection.	30% of all babies born to mothers with AIDS will die.	No cure.	Sexual self-control before and after marriage

† Babies can contract STDs during pregnancy or birth from the mother.

fatigue, nausea, vomiting, and diarrhea. Later symptoms include abdominal pain, a yellowing of the whites of the eyes and skin, grayish stools, and dark urine. About 15 to 20 percent of those with hepatitis B may also experience temporary arthritis-like symptoms.

About 10 percent of those infected in the United States go on to develop a chronic, or long-lasting, form of the disease. Such people are at risk for cirrhosis and cancer of the liver. They may also infect others. The NIAID estimates that there are about 1.5 million chronic carriers in the United States and about three hundred million worldwide. This does not include newly infected people, who are also infectious.

HBV is transmitted through body fluids: blood and blood products, semen and vaginal fluids, and saliva. Sexual intercourse, blood transfusions, and other exchanges of body fluids—through broken skin or shared drug needles—can transmit the disease.

All pregnant women should take a blood test for hepatitis B. They might have the virus and infect their babies without knowing it.

Hepatitis B is one of the few sexually transmitted diseases for which there is a vaccine.

OTHER STDs

In addition to the seven sexually transmitted diseases we've discussed, others include: vaginitis (inflammation of the vagina), pubic lice (crabs), scabies, molluscum contagiosum, chancroid, lymphogranuloma venereum, granuloma inguinale, cytomegalovirus infections, amebiasis, mycoplasma infections, and streptococcal infections. The list of germs that can be passed through sexual contact continues to grow.

The surest way to prevent STDs is to abstain from sex until marriage and to remain completely monogamous thereafter. Changing sex partners over time—known as mutual or serial monogamy—does not protect a person from contracting a sexually transmitted disease. Serial monogamy carries the same risk as having sex with all of one's partners in the same night.

CONDOMS

On December 17, 1995, seventeen-year-old Meggan died of Kaposi's sarcoma, a cancer that afflicts many AIDS sufferers. She had sex only twice in her life—both times with a condom. Although most cases take longer, Meggan contracted HIV, developed AIDS, and died within two years.

To those who knew her, Meggan was a thoughtful, loving person. "She was so ashamed of her disease that she could never bring herself to tell me she had it," said a close friend.

The friend later received a letter that Meggan wrote before she died, describing her thoughts and feelings. Meggan's parents said that their daughter did not want the girl to remember Meggan as a dying AIDS victim, but as her best friend.

"Finally I talked to the guy who gave her the disease," the friend said. "He didn't know that he was infected at the time he gave it to her and told me repeatedly how sorry he was for 'killing' her." Although he was HIV positive, the boy hadn't yet developed AIDS symptoms. He felt bad that he was alive and Meggan was gone.

"It doesn't happen very often that the person who passes on this [disease] lives to feel the pain and remorse of seeing the results of their carelessness," the friend said. "But he lives each day knowing that sooner or later he will be joining her. He isn't as good at hiding it from the world as Meggan was."[39]

Many people think that using a condom is a way to have safe sex. But Meggan's story forces us to ask: How safe are condoms?

The answer depends on what you want to be safe *from*. It also depends on the condition of the condoms (condoms exposed to excessive heat or crushed in a wallet can become defective). So, too, it depends on who is using the condoms and how experienced they are.

For example, let's say you wanted to protect yourself from pregnancy. On average, about 16 percent of all couples in the United States who rely on condoms for birth control get pregnant

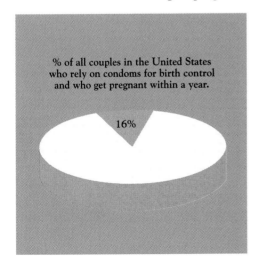

% of all couples in the United States who rely on condoms for birth control and who get pregnant within a year.

16%

within a year.[40] Worldwide, the very lowest one-year failure rate in a large study is 4.2 percent. The people who participated in that study, however, were highly motivated married couples ages twenty-five to thirty-nine.[41]

But what about STDs, the topic of this chapter? As before, the answer depends on the condition of the condoms, who is using the condoms, and how experienced they are. It also depends on the particular STD. But all in all, condoms provide even less protection against STDs than they do against pregnancy.

There are three important reasons why this is so. For one thing, the germs that cause STDs have a much larger target to aim at than sperm cells. In order to make a woman pregnant, a sperm cell must find and fertilize *a single cell*—the egg. That's like finding a needle in a haystack. The germs that cause STDs, on the other hand, need only find a moist internal membrane to launch an infection. Some germs don't even need that: they can infect you if they land on your skin. These germs include the herpes simplex virus, human papillomavirus, and the bacterium that causes syphilis (*Treponema pallidum*).

Another reason why condoms are less effective at preventing disease is that germs can reproduce. If a sperm cell escapes from a condom, it may fertilize the woman's egg, but it cannot form other sperm cells. Viruses, bacteria, and parasites, however, do not have this limitation. If they escape from a condom and invade the body's defenses, they can reproduce, making more of their kind.

A final reason why condoms are less effective at preventing disease than they are at preventing pregnancy is that a woman can get pregnant only three to five days during each month. But a man or woman can contract an STD any time—twenty-four hours a day, every day of the year.

The degree of risk depends on the disease. For example, herpes simplex virus, human papillomavirus, and *Treponema pallidum* can all be spread by skin-to-skin contact. If your partner has sores from one of these diseases, and your skin comes into contact with them, you too can become infected. The same may be true if your skin comes into contact with an infected person's sexual fluids. In both cases, a condom would be completely useless.

Jenny, a twenty-two-year-old college student, visited her gynecologist complaining of a small growth on her vulva. The doctor took a biopsy which indicated a precancerous lesion. If Jenny had not seen the growth or sought treatment, she would eventually have faced cancer surgery.

"But how could this happen?" Jenny asked her doctor. "I've been so careful. We used a condom every time!"

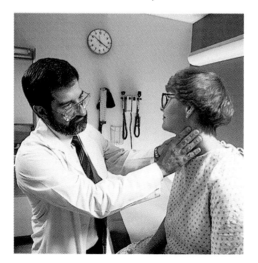

"Except with Steve," she admitted. "He was the first—but we were both virgins." After that, Jenny said, she had sex with four other partners.

The growth on Jenny's vulva was caused by the human papillomavirus and started when semen from one of her boyfriends spilled onto her after they had sex—even though they "used a condom every time." Condoms did not protect Jenny from getting HPV.

Even with diseases that aren't spread by skin contact, however, condoms do not provide complete protection. Studies show that the risk of gonorrhea, for example, may be reduced by about 50 to 75 percent.[42] The risk of HIV infection seems to be reduced by 57 to 80 percent.[43] The risk for chlamydia does not seem to be reduced at all.[44]

Some of these percentages may seem pretty large, making it sound as if condoms can greatly reduce your risk of infection. But even with such reductions, you still run a sizeable risk of becoming infected. Unless you are in a strictly monogamous relationship with an uninfected partner, that risk increases each time you have sex. In fact, even if you reduce your risk by as much as 80 percent, by the time you have had sex five times you will have the same level of risk as someone who has had sex once with no protection at all.

What's more, you don't get to choose what disease your partner might have. Even if a condom could eliminate all risk of contracting an HIV infection, that won't do you any good if your partner has the human papillomavirus.

Perhaps the best indicator of risk, though, is what experts would do if they had to rely on condoms for protection. A speaker posed the following question

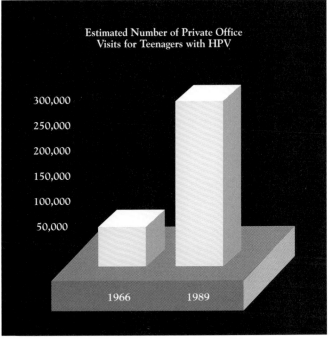

Estimated Number of Private Office Visits for Teenagers with HPV

300,000
250,000
200,000
150,000
100,000
50,000

1966   1989

to a group of sex educators: "Imagine that you were approached by the man or woman of your dreams, the person you thought would be the best sex partner for you in all the world. If this person offered himself or herself to you but said, 'I want you to know that I have AIDS,' would you have sex with that person, using only a condom for protection?"

At first no one raised a hand. Finally one person raised his hand slowly.

The speaker then asked the group, "Why, if you are unwilling to trust condoms, are you encouraging students throughout the country to rely on them for protection against AIDS and many other diseases?"[45]

According to the surgeon general's report on AIDS, "If you're young and you haven't yet achieved a mutually faithful monogamous relationship... then you should by all means take the best possible precautions against disease by abstaining. Period. That is my advice...and I don't think there's any better advice you can give."[46]

The only sure way to avoid getting STDs, including AIDS, is to wait until you have established a mutually faithful monogamous relationship. Monogamy is defined in *Merriam Webster's Collegiate Dictionary* as being married to one person for life. The only place to find such a relationship is within marriage. Marriage is the healthiest setting for sexual activity, particularly if you and your spouse have both exercised sexual self-control until marriage.

Persons who engage in risk-taking behaviors, such as drug abuse or sexual activity outside marriage, should stop. The more risks they take, the more likely they are to become infected. Young people who have engaged in unhealthy behaviors but decide to regain sexual self-control should consider seeing a doctor. A doctor's encouragement may strengthen their decision to regain self-control. Also, a medical checkup is important because STDs have serious long-term consequences if not detected in time. Finally, a clean bill of health frees you to enjoy life.

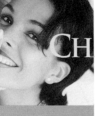

SAY YES TO A DISEASE-FREE LIFESTYLE

Teens who practice sexual self-control reap tremendous benefits both now and in the future. In particular, they experience a disease-free lifestyle—a lifestyle free from the harmful consequences of STDs. Sexual self-control frees you from many negative and psychologically painful experiences. These include:

FREEDOM FROM EMBARRASSMENT, GUILT, WORRY, AND SHAME

Embarrassment usually results from contracting an STD. Ask yourself if you would want all your friends to know about an STD you have contracted.

Guilt comes from realizing that you shouldn't have been sexually active and that being sexually active caused your STD. Would you want to tell your parents about an STD you have contracted? Why would it be difficult to tell them?

One psychiatrist observed, "The number of herpes patients has decreased since 1982. However, the herpes patients I see [now] suffer intense guilt feelings and feelings that they are unclean and dirty. Herpes patients fear the most that they will not find a partner or someone who wants them."[47]

Worry can arise from wondering if the person you are dating has an STD. Do you know how many other sexual partners that person has had? Can you be sure someone does not have an STD just because he or she says so?

On the other hand, can you be sure that you yourself don't have an STD? Many STDs go undetected and have no signs or symptoms. If you've been sexually active, how can you be sure you don't have an STD? And if you have an STD, how can you be sure you won't spread it to others?

Shame may also result from contracting an STD. You probably wouldn't want to discuss this with your family at the dinner table or brag about it to your neighbors. Why wouldn't you?

FREEDOM FROM CONSTANT MEDICAL CHECKUPS

Most STDs go unnoticed and undetected until symptoms occur. If not diagnosed and treated in time, many STDs can lead to serious complications. Short of a doctor's visit, you can't be sure if someone has an STD. Thus, when people tell you they don't have an STD or have not had an STD, there is no guarantee that they are telling the truth. They may not even know they have an STD. Bottom line: Every time people engage in premarital sex, they risk getting an STD, including AIDS.

FREEDOM FROM DAMAGING MAJOR BODY ORGANS

Several STDs can leave the body organs impaired. PID can destroy a woman's ability to have a baby. The heart and parts of the reproductive, nervous, and immune systems in both sexes can be damaged by STDs.

FREEDOM FROM TELLING YOUR PARENTS YOU HAVE AN STD

Most parents want their children to come to them with their problems. They want to know if their children are sick—even if that sickness is an STD. At first, parents may be disappointed, hurt, or shocked. But they are usually the best ally adolescents have in regaining good health. Most adults know the medical field better than teenagers do—adults have used medical services over a longer period of time. If you have an STD, let your parents help. Try also to understand how they feel. And don't be too hard on yourself: unwise decisions do not make bad people.

Sexual self-control doesn't just free you from the negative consequences of STDs, but it also enables you to enjoy the following positive freedoms:

FREEDOM TO LIVE

Poor decisions can produce irreversible consequences, even death. Fortunately, you don't have to keep on making poor decisions. You can start making good decisions right now. If you are addicted to drugs or alcohol, get help at a rehabilitation center. An out-of-wedlock pregnancy can be very traumatic. If you are pregnant and not married, find help at a crisis pregnancy center. If you've been having premarital sex and want to stop, find someone you trust and who will hold you accountable.

FREEDOM TO KNOW YOU ARE HEALTHY

According to the Centers for Disease Control in Atlanta, three million teenagers suffer from STDs annually. This number represents only the three million teens who *know* they have an STD.[48]

Consider the following facts about women:

- About 80 percent of women show no signs of gonorrhea.
- About 70 percent of women show no signs of chlamydia.
- Numerous cervical cancer cases go undetected by Pap smears.

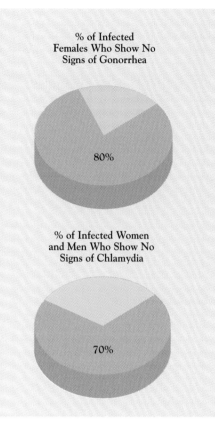

% of Infected Females Who Show No Signs of Gonorrhea

80%

% of Infected Women and Men Who Show No Signs of Chlamydia

70%

Many diseases can lie dormant within the body and go undiagnosed and undetected; but the disease can still be spreading in a person's body and be spread to a sexual partner. Herpes, for instance, can be contagious even when no lesions are visible. Sexual self-control is the best way to lead a disease-free lifestyle and remain healthy.

FREEDOM TO ESTABLISH PHYSICALLY HEALTHY DATING RELATIONSHIPS

If you are not married, sexual abstinence is the only way to avoid risking an STD. Risk-taking begins when an individual engages in unhealthy dating habits. A person can acquire an STD

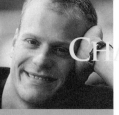

through one experience of sexual intercourse. Even sexual intimacy without intercourse can allow an STD to be transmitted.

For instance, studies have shown that STDs can be transmitted by open-mouth or "French" kissing. One study examined the relationship between passionate kissing and the transmission of the AIDS virus. Forty-five heterosexual couples were asked to collect saliva immediately before and after passionate kissing. Ninety-one percent had blood in their saliva after passionate kissing. Researchers concluded that "the results of this study indicate that passionate kissing cannot be considered protective safe sex [against] the transmission of the AIDS virus."[49]

A disease-free lifestyle includes healthy dating habits. Healthy dating habits help young adults establish healthy relationships. You can be proud of healthy dating habits—they pay off.

FREEDOM TO KNOW YOU ARE NOT INFECTING YOUR FUTURE SPOUSE

Many people choose immediate gratification over future rewards. By engaging in premarital sex, you sacrifice your future well-being for immediate pleasure.

The decision to engage in premarital sex seriously affects other people, both physically and emotionally. Along with you and your partner, these other people include your parents and family, your partner's parents and family, future spouses, and future unborn children.

If you love your partner and plan to marry, you do not want to infect the person you love with an STD. By exercising sexual self-control before marriage, you can be certain that you will not infect your future spouse with an STD. Teenagers may make unhealthy decisions in high school and suffer the consequences in the future. But future rewards are built on delaying immediate gratification.

FREEDOM TO HAVE HEALTHY BABIES

STDs can prevent a woman from having a child, either by making her infertile, or by adversely affecting her pregnancy (as happens in an ectopic, or tubal, pregnancy). But even if she is able to conceive and give birth, an infected mother can still pass the disease to her child.

Exercising self-control before marriage improves the chances of having healthy children within marriage. Although having children may be the farthest thing from your mind now, it will become a very real possibility in the future.

A television commercial depicts a married woman who has a wonderful husband and home but is unable to have children. She tells the audience she cannot have children because an STD has left her sterile. She explains that she never understood how serious STDs were.

The only sure defense against STDs is sexual abstinence or a completely monogamous relationship—marriage—between two uninfected partners who do not use intravenous drugs. Any other choice puts you and your partner at risk for all of the diseases mentioned in this chapter.

1. Condoms have a one-in-six failure rate. Would you skydive with a parachute that had a one-in-six chance of *not* opening? When is a one-in-six failure rate acceptable? When is it unacceptable?

2. People who have premarital sex usually do not marry their partners. Thus, when you have premarital sex with someone, you probably are having sex with someone else's future husband or wife. How would you feel if your future spouse contracted an STD from someone else? What if your future spouse became sterile because of it?

3. Why do young people who contract an STD sometimes feel "dirty" and think "no one will want me"?

4. Many STDs go undetected and have no signs or symptoms. Would you marry someone who had been sexually active with other people but refused a medical checkup?

5. Complications of STDs can lead to sterility. Is sterility worth risking with someone you won't end up marrying?

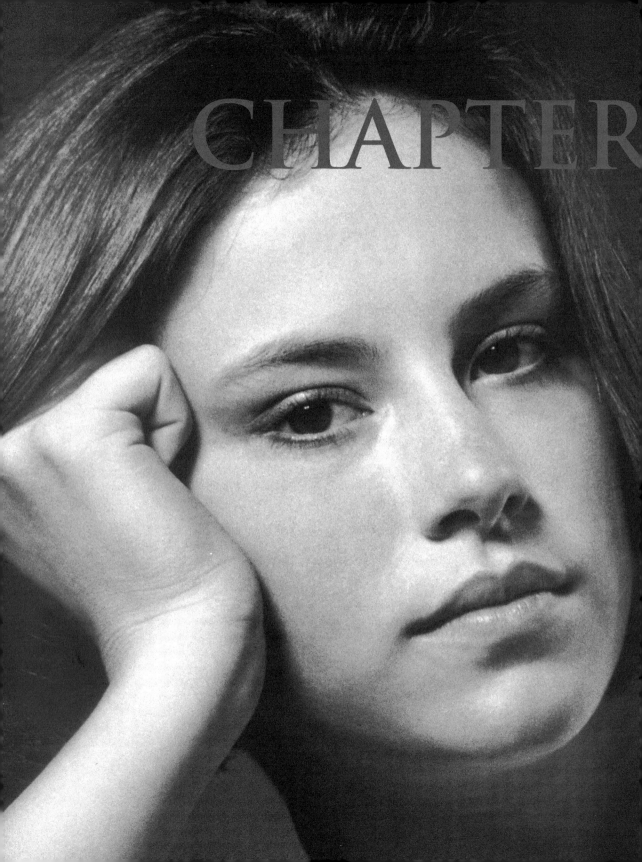

Having premarital sex is risky. Even with birth control, there are still risks. *Many young people do not think about STDs or getting pregnant when they have sex before marriage. The sad thing is that they should because it might happen to them. Everyone always thinks that bad things will happen to other people; they never think anything bad will happen to them. But it does.*

RISKY BUSINESS: PREGNANCY

-A high school senior, West Springfield, Virginia

When Katrina Mroczek, of Grand Rapids, Michigan, told her father she was sexually active, he took her to the gynecologist's office for the birth-control device Norplant. But they were too late. The doctor told Katrina, age fifteen, that she was already pregnant.

Dazed, she watched as tears fell from her father's eyes. He had had high hopes for his beautiful daughter's future: a college education, a successful career, travel, a home. But in an instant his hopes were shattered—just as his dreams for his own life had been many years before.

Stanley Mroczek had dreamed of joining the navy and traveling to far-off places. But then his girlfriend told him she was pregnant. A young woman with plans of her own—to become a nurse—Tammy Billiau quit school and, soon after Katrina was born, married Stanley. He started working in a factory, and in a short time two more children were born to the young couple.

Stanley eventually lost his job and, with little education, had a hard time securing another one. The work he found didn't pay the bills: the electricity was turned off, the car was repossessed, and the couple ended up applying for welfare. After several years Stanley attended school and took a position as a

But the strain of poverty had left its mark on the couple. They divorced when Katrina was twelve.

Stanley Mroczek hadn't wanted his daughter to suffer in the same way.

But Katrina was optimistic about her pregnancy. "I'll be OK," she told her father. "I'll still finish high school and get a good job."

She expected the baby's father, Doug Jones, who had also dropped out of high school, to help.

Jurnee was born on April 22, 1995. She quickly outgrew her new baby clothes. The thrift store was the only place Katrina could afford to shop. Jurnee was often sick and spent time in the hospital with a blood infection when she was ten months old.

Life wasn't going the way Katrina expected. Devoting most of her time and energy to the baby, she got behind in school. She and Doug had problems, and he moved in with his mother. He saw Katrina only occasionally and bought

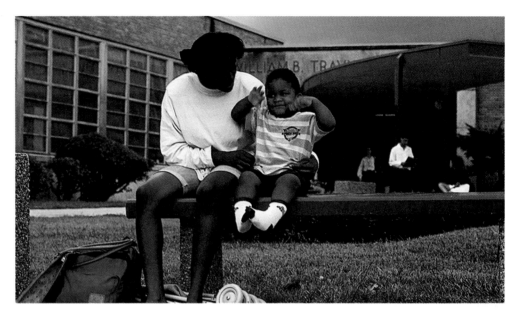

Katrina and her daughter now live with her mother. Although she still hopes to finish high school someday, she's earned only three of the twenty credits she needs to graduate.

"I wish she could have learned from my and Tammy's mistakes," said Stanley Mroczek. "Katrina has a fantasy world and sees great things ahead, but I just see another welfare mom."[1]

Things often don't work out the way people think they will. Here are some of the harsh realities.

A single mother has a heavy burden of responsibilities, but a single *teenage* mother has even more. If she doesn't finish high school, her chances for a higher education are slim to none, and her hopes for a good-paying job seldom materialize. Parenting adds an even greater weight.

Family researcher Barbara Dafoe Whitehead observes, "Half the single mothers in the United States live below the poverty line. (Currently, one out of ten married couples with children is

poor.) Many others live on the edge of poverty. Even single mothers who are far from poor are likely to experience persistent economic insecurity."[2]

According to William A. Galston, former deputy assistant to the president for domestic public policy, Americans who graduate from high school, reach age twenty, and marry before having their first child have only an 8 percent chance of their child being raised in poverty. If, however, they don't follow these three steps before having their first child, the risk that the child will grow up in poverty increases to 79 percent.[3]

Remarking on these statistics, syndicated newspaper columnist William Raspberry notes, "It's hard for children to foresee the consequences of premature sex or to imagine that their delightful little babies can turn into anchors that hold them in poverty."[4]

That's not to say that children are a burden—to be disposed of at will. Pregnancy is not a disease to be "cured" by medical technology. Indeed, parenthood is demanding precisely because each child is so valuable. But until you're in a position to meet that responsibility fully, you're better off avoiding any risk of pregnancy.

WHAT ARE THE CHOICES?

More than a million teenage girls, most of them unmarried, become pregnant each year. What's more, there are about 350,000 new unmarried teen mothers each year.[5] When a girl gets pregnant, both the boy and the girl become parents. As parents, they both share the responsibility of caring for the unborn child.

An important part of sharing that responsibility is realizing that children grow best when their own father and mother live with them full-time. Sociologist David Popenoe summarizes decades of research when he says, "On the whole, for children, two-parent families are preferable to single-parent families and stepfamilies."[6]

The consequences of unmarried sex, however, fall mainly on the mother and her child. Pregnancy and childbirth often bring major economic and lifestyle changes for the mother. The child is also affected—not just at birth, but from the moment of conception (see sidebar "Some Facts about Prenatal Development"). Nutrition, drugs, alcohol, and tobacco can all have a profound impact on the developing child. So can many diseases.

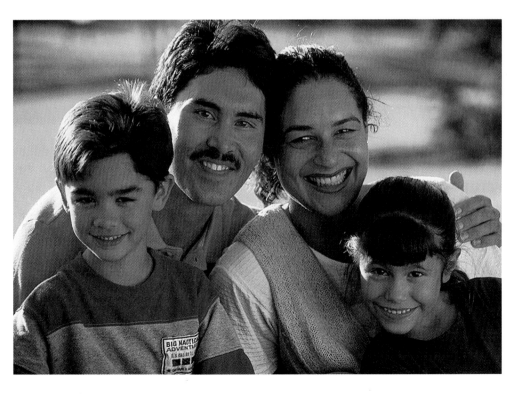

SOME FACTS ABOUT PRENATAL DEVELOPMENT

New life is created at the moment the father's sperm unites with the mother's egg. Other scientific facts regarding life in the mother's womb include:

- Within four to eight days of conception, the fertilized egg attaches itself to the mother's womb.
- By that time, the child's sex has already been determined.
- At seventeen days from conception, the child's own blood cells, distinct from the mother's, are present.
- At nineteen days, the baby's eyes start to form.
- By the twenty-fifth day, the child's heart begins beating.
- In the fourth to fifth week, the small unborn child looks distinctly human, yet the child's mother still may not know that she is pregnant.
- By the sixth week, the baby's brainwaves can be detected with an electroencephalograph (EEG), the fingers begin to develop, and the baby has nostrils.
- By eight weeks, the beginnings of all the baby's key body parts are present, although they are not completely developed. The baby has ears, fingers, and toes.
- Between eight and ten weeks, the baby begins making small, random movements, which the mother cannot yet feel.
- By ten weeks, the baby's heartbeat can be detected. By this time, fingernails are developing; and the baby can squint, swallow, move his or her tongue, and make a tight fist.
- Brain cells are being produced at an average rate of 250,000 per minute, and upon completion will number over 100 billion.

From about ten or twelve weeks until the end of pregnancy, development is mainly fine-tuning and further growth.

Young women who did not plan to become pregnant usually need medical care, counseling, housing, financial aid, schooling and job assistance, and legal aid. Those needs vary with the mother's age, maturity, health, economic status, and relationships with family, friends, and the baby's father.

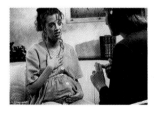

During pregnancy a young unmarried mother must ask herself:

- Will I eat properly?
- Will I get the proper amount of exercise and rest for my baby's health?
- Will I smoke, even though smoking will affect my unborn baby?
- Will I use drugs, including alcohol, even though drugs will affect my unborn baby?
- Will I see a doctor frequently while I'm pregnant—to get adequate prenatal care?

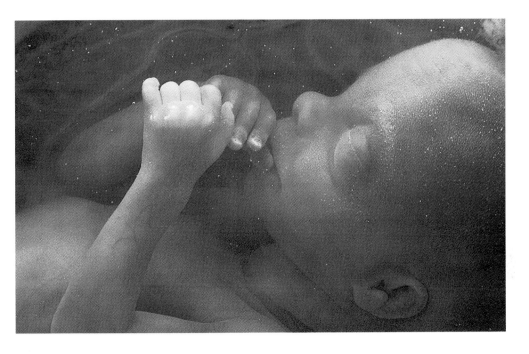

The father and the mother must ask themselves:

- Will we get married?
- How will we provide for our child?
- Who will raise our child? Will we raise our child, or will someone else?
- Should we place our child for adoption?

Do a teen mother and a teen father know what's right in each of these choices? Do they care enough about what's right to make the right moral choices, thinking not only of themselves, but also of what's best for their child?

Pregnancy centers help teens and young adults answer these questions, and they can also help with many of their physical, emotional, and legal needs. The kinds of help they offer include food, clothing, medical attention, counseling, babysitting, and even a place to live. To contact a center near you, look under "Abortion Alternatives" in the Yellow Pages.

Teen pregnancy affects everyone involved—the father, the mother, and their respective families. Under current law, however, the mother makes the final choice between keeping the child, giving the child up for adoption, or aborting the child. Each choice carries serious consequences.

KEEPING THE CHILD

Kate was fourteen when she met Dave. He was well-liked, especially by the students who drank alcohol and smoked marijuana. Kate enjoyed being with Dave. After several months of steady dating, the couple decided to have sex. Dave used condoms, but Kate got pregnant anyway.

She decided to keep and raise her daughter. She finished high school but felt awkward while she was there. Some of her friends shunned her while others said they envied her.

Nine years later, Kate and her daughter, Michelle, were still living with her parents. She worked during the day and attended night classes at a local college. "I missed out on a lot of the fun of being a teenager," the young mother said.

Saving sex for marriage allows teens to be teens instead of throwing them into adult situations that rob them of their adolescent years.

Remember Tanya and Katrina? Both girls decided to keep their children. As unmarried mothers, they faced hard challenges, such as having to drop out of school and work two jobs. Single mothers and their children have a much higher chance of living in poverty. Expectant single mothers need to be realistic about the challenges they will face when deciding what to do. They should ask themselves not only what is best for them, but what is best for the child.

ADOPTION

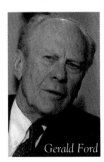

Gerald Ford

What do Dave Thomas, founder of Wendy's Restaurants; Gerald Ford, former president of the United States; and Scott Hamilton, Olympic gold-medal figure skater, have in common? All three were adopted.[7] Amie Beth Dickinson, former Miss Alabama, was also adopted.

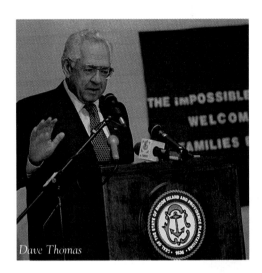

Dave Thomas

Three decades ago, more than 90 percent of unmarried teenage girls who gave birth placed their babies for adoption. Today, however, despite the benefits that adoption offers to teen parents and their child, only 2 to 3 percent place their babies with adoptive parents.[8]

Many counselors believe that adoption is the best choice for unmarried pregnant women. Even so, almost 40 percent of teen pregnancy counseling does not mention adoption, primarily because few counselors think teens want to know about it.[9]

Research indicates that unmarried birth mothers who choose adoption for their children are less likely to be poor, less likely to receive public assistance, and more likely to finish high school than unmarried birth mothers who keep their children.[10]

According to the National Family Growth Survey, adopted children are much less likely to live in poverty than children living with their never-married birth mothers. Adoptive mothers are usually older and have a better education than never-married birth mothers.[11]

A lot of people want to adopt. More than a million couples in the United States face infertility problems and will never be able to conceive. These couples apply and wait for the fifty thousand children who become available each year for adoption. This means that for each adoptable child at least twenty couples are waiting and hoping to adopt a child.[12]

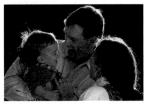

It takes maturity and unselfishness for a teen mother and father to give their child up for adoption when they know they can't raise the child properly. They make that hard decision out of love for their child. A natural bond typically forms as the mother carries her baby inside her. The bond strengthens when the mother sees her baby at birth. Although placing a baby for adoption is always difficult, it may be the most loving and unselfish decision a young mother can make.

The involvement of the baby's father in decision-making is also important, even though it can be difficult and emotional for the baby's mother. He can play a positive and important role in their lives. His needs and feelings should be considered, and he should understand the adoption alternative.

By choosing adoption, the natural parents are putting the child's interests first. Adoption can provide a child with a full-time mother and father, financial security, physical health and well-being, and better opportunities for the future.

Adoption also makes it possible for teens to stay in school and learn skills and qualities they will need as maturing adults. Too many teens think they can raise a child successfully. But adoption may be the wiser choice, resulting in a better future for both the mother and her child.

Nikki faced such a challenge. She was a high school senior preparing for college. She was in love with Matthew and decided at the end of the school year to have sex with him. After one time of intercourse, she became pregnant.

Nikki's parents advised her to abort the baby. She chose instead to give birth and find a good family to parent the child. After her little girl was born, she placed her in a home with a couple who could not have children of their own.

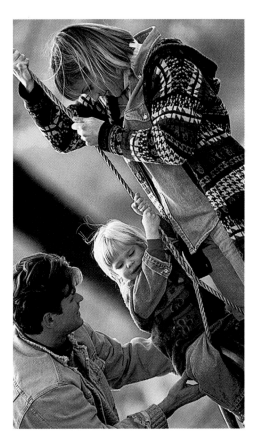

Nikki entered college and later went on to graduate school. After ten years she earned a master's degree in social work.

In the past two decades the concept of open adoption has become more accepted. This allows the birth mother, the birth father, and the adoptive parents to communicate in various ways, such as sending one-way letters through a middle person; trading letters and pictures; or even meeting in person.

In the following letter Kristin, a young birth mother, explains to the adoptive parents why she gave up her daughter and how hard it was to do so. She also describes her pregnancy and delivery, and expresses a desire to keep in touch with the parents and eventually with her daughter. Kristin assures them of her love and that she will leave those decisions to them.

Dear Beautiful People,

I just found out today that you received my baby. I don't know you and I don't know if our paths will ever cross in life, but I want you to know that I am eternally grateful to you, and I love you both with all my heart. It is really strange. We are so distant, but yet I feel so close to you....

Giving up this baby was the hardest thing in my life that I have ever done, but it was because I have loved her so much that I made my decision. I want her to have the kind of raising that I had, two loving parents that could provide her with the spiritual, emotional, and material needs that are involved with raising a child. The main thing being two parents that love her, which is something I couldn't provide by myself. Don't get me wrong, I could smother her with love, but there is so much more to it than that, that

I know you can provide for her. I hope you don't mind me referring to her as "my" baby, I realize I gave her up legally, and she is yours, but I do have maternal feelings toward her. I hope you understand what I'm trying to say....

When she was born I went to see her and got to hold her. I thought she was beautiful—I hope you do! It really hit me hard, the fact of what I was doing—as I was holding her, looking at her and thinking about her—I started crying. It hurt so much, but I knew what I wanted and what she needed. Even as young as I am, I realize that raising a child is a hard thing to do....

I'd like to keep in touch with you and you with me—but only if you want. I don't want you to feel I'm imposing, it's just that I'd like to know how your family is growing together. Also, I'd like to ask you to send me a picture of her in a few months—I'm curious to see what she looks like then, but I'm leaving the decision up to you. Whatever you feel best....

If you have any questions—just let me know. I'm keeping close contact with the agency, and am looking forward to hearing from you. God bless you and your family and may you have a happy and prosperous life.

Take care!

I Love You[13]

Today Kristin is a nurse's aide. She looks forward to finishing college, future marriage, and future children. Kristin remembers her firstborn daughter as much today as when she wrote this letter.

Sandra, a nineteen-year-old birth mother, wrote the following letter to her child explaining her reasons for choosing adoption.

Dear Daughter,

I'm writing this letter almost one year after I had you because I feel like it is something that I must do before too long. I want you to know my reasons for giving you up and tell you that you are now and will be forever in my thoughts. There were many times that I would change my mind, but in the end my decision was the best for everyone all the way around.

I want you to know that if your birth father and I could have provided for you everything necessary, we would have done so. When I say provided for you, I mean everything needed to raise a child including love for each other, which was not there. I don't think I was old enough to take the responsibility of raising a child either. I am sure that if your birth father and I loved each other as much as we love you, we could have done it. However, it wasn't that way between us. We thought we did, but when it came to talking about the rest of our lives, I really don't think it was there.

I am sure now that you are happy and have the most wonderful parents ever dreamed of. They are warm, loving people and I admire them very much. I know you will grow into a beautiful person and have a great life.

I cannot put down into writing the way I feel about you. Now that a year has passed by, my life has gone on and the memories that I have of you are stored in a special place in my heart. Your birth father and I have remained friends and we both hope that we may see you someday. I hope your feelings will be the same and you can understand our reasons for placing you for adoption.

Love always,
Your Birth Mother[14]

Unlike Kristin and Sandra, Allison understood what it was like to be adopted. She, too, was adopted and recalls growing up "always knowing I was adopted." She and her husband adopted a little boy. Allison wrote the following letter to her son's birth mother to introduce herself and reassure her of their love for her son. She tells the birth mother how much she admires her courage and respects her for doing what she felt was best for her son—and how grateful she is for that decision.

To the Birth Mother of Our Son,

First, I would like to thank you for the very beautiful letters you sent to us and our son. I know that someday they will be very meaningful to him and will help him to understand his adoption.

I would like to tell you a little about myself. I, too, was adopted. I was born in San Antonio. However, since my Dad was in the service, I spent most of my growing years all over the world. Our family is extremely close-knit. I have a brother and sister, also adopted. Our parents are truly wonderful people and we have always felt very loved and very secure. My mother and father were very open and honest with us about the circumstances of our adoption. I never felt that I was unwanted and I know that my son will understand why you could not care for him....

I have so many feelings I would like to express to you. Compassion—I know your decision to give your baby up for adoption was a difficult one. I admire your courage and respect you for doing what you felt to be in the best interest of your baby. I am extremely grateful to you for giving us a beautiful son for our own....

What else can I tell you? From the very first moment that I held him, I loved him and felt he was mine. Each day that I wake up and look at him, I can hardly believe it. Our love for him grows stronger each day, and we enjoy watching him develop.

I have saved all the information and papers regarding his adoption and birth to place in a scrapbook. I intend to put it in storybook form, so that he will have his own little story. I hope that we will be able to make him feel as secure in our love for him as my parents made me feel.

I could go on and on, but there are really not enough appropriate words to express my feelings. I love our beautiful son and I will have a special place in my heart for the woman who made my dreams become a reality.
Thank you.[15]

Birth fathers are affected by adoption as well. Russell, a nineteen-year-old birth father, expressed his feelings for his daughter in the following letter. He is sorry that he and his daughter won't spend their lives together, but he does not regret placing her for adoption. He knows that it is best for her. He explains that he and her mother loved her very much, but they did not love each other and could not provide a loving home for her.

Dear Daughter,
I want to start this letter by telling you how sorry I am, although I am not sorry for placing you for adoption; I am only sorry that we cannot spend our lives together. Although I only really knew you for a day, I will miss you, and I will always have you in my heart.
The situation between your birth

mother and me was that we both loved you very much, but we didn't love each other. We could give you love but not a home. A child needs a home with two people who care and love that child together. This your birth mother and I could not provide…. Our decision was a difficult one, because it is not easy to give up one so dear. The only way we could do this was because we knew that through adoption you would get the chance you really deserve to grow up healthy and happy. I pray that you will forgive us and understand why we placed you for adoption.

By the time you read this letter you will have grown enough to hopefully know why we did what we did. Your birth mother and I love you very much. I hope this letter will help you as much as it has helped me. I shall never forget you, and I will always have the hope that someday we will meet so that we can satisfy both our curiosity, and see what each other is really like. Daughter, have a wonderful life, and I Love You.
Love Always,
Birth Father[16]

Adoption is a hard decision to make, one that requires strong character. If you are considering that choice, you should not feel pressured. Ask for a reasonable amount of time after your baby is born to confirm your decision. And don't be afraid to ask for counseling and support.

If you are pregnant and are considering adoption, there are many places you can turn. One good source of counseling and information is a local crisis pregnancy center. You can see if there are centers near you by looking in the Yellow Pages under "Abortion Alternatives." The following organizations can also help you:

Adoption Options
1724 N. Burnside, #7
Gonzales, LA 70737
504-644-1033

Adoptive Families of America
3333 Highway 100
North Minneapolis, MN 55422
612-535-4829

AIDS Orphan Adoption Project
c/o National Council for Adoption
1930 17th Street, NW
Washington, DC 20009
800-333-NCFA

Bethany Christian Services
901 Eastern Avenue, NE
Grand Rapids, MI 49501
800-BETHANY

Down's Syndrome Adoption Exchange
56 Midchester Avenue
White Plains, NY 10606
914-428-1236

Gladney Center
2300 Hemphill
Fort Worth, TX 76110
817-922-6000
800-GLADNEY

National Adoption Center
1500 Walnut Street
Philadelphia, PA 19102
215-735-9988
800-TO-ADOPT

National Council for Adoption
1930 17th Street, NW
Washington, DC 20009
202-328-1200
800-333-NCFA

National Resource Center for Special-Needs Adoption
16250 Northland Drive
Suite 120
Southfield, MI 48075
810-443-7080

The Nurturing Network
910 Main Street
Suite 360
Boise, ID 83702
800-TNN-4MOM

ABORTION

My first sexual encounter was at the age of fifteen with my boyfriend, who was two years older than I. We were at a party, and, after a week or two of dating, I fell for the "If you really love me" line.

We didn't use any protection—except withdrawal, which is no protection at all—the first time or for months thereafter. I don't know why we didn't.... Eight months later...I got pregnant.

I was sixteen then, a junior in high school. I had an abortion. Although we continued dating another year, it devastated me and our relationship. Only now have I begun to understand the enormity of my abortion and am beginning to forgive myself.[17]

After years of being sexually active, the young woman who wrote these words became a "secondary virgin" at the age of twenty-three. She chose to remain abstinent until marriage.

Abortion often seems like the quickest, easiest way to resolve a crisis pregnancy. The truth is, however, it is much more complex.

Since abortion was legalized nationwide in 1973, over 30 million abortions have taken place in America. According to the Alan Guttmacher Institute, about 1.4 million abortions took place in 1994.[18] In its report *Sex and America's Teenagers*, the Guttmacher Institute notes that "half of the more than 1 million pregnancies among adolescent women each year end in birth; a third end in abortion. Most of the births are unintended."[19] Altogether, teens comprise almost one-fourth of all abortions performed each year.[20]

The operation has risks. Abortion is almost universally fatal to the unborn child, of course. But the procedure itself also carries risks for both the mother and father. The father faces emotional risks, while the mother faces physical ones as well.

Three months following his father's unexpected death, Peter, an eighteen-year-old who worked at a gas station, shot and killed himself. At the time of the suicide Peter had been depressed, said his closest friend, because his girlfriend had aborted their baby. Peter believed they had conceived the child on the same day his father died. He was expecting a son and was already forming images of the baby in his mind; he planned to name the baby after his father. Losing the child and all that the child stood for was too much for Peter.[21]

The emotional consequences of an abortion can be long-lasting. A woman, age seventy-five, lived in a nursing home. Those who passed near her room thought she was psychotic. They heard her mumble repeatedly: "I killed my baby! I killed my baby!"

Sixty years earlier, the woman had undergone an abortion. She had never gotten over her loss or her guilt.[22]

The trauma of abortion crosses cultures. Akiko, a Japanese college student studying in the United States, was referred to a psychiatrist for what was diagnosed as premenstrual syndrome. Her symptoms were actually brought on by the monthly anniversary of her abortion. The staff in her dormitory reported that each month, for a day or two, Akiko would isolate herself in her room and weep, not coming out even for classes or meals.

As it turned out, the day before Akiko left Japan she had undergone an abortion. She came to America to study early childhood education. The first classes she took were about prenatal development. As she watched a film depicting life in the uterus, she realized for the first time what stage of development her own child had reached at the time of her abortion, just weeks earlier. After that, on the monthly anniversary of her abortion, guilt and profound sadness filled Akiko, but she could not share her feelings with anyone.

In working with Akiko, the psychiatrist discovered how Japanese women handle their grief following an abortion. They ask for memorial services to be held in honor of the children lost through abortion. Parents may even rent statues of children from Buddhist temples to offer prayers on behalf of the child. These statues can be seen in cemeteries throughout Japan.[23]

The trauma of abortion also affects medical professionals. Barbara, an experienced nurse in an intensive care unit

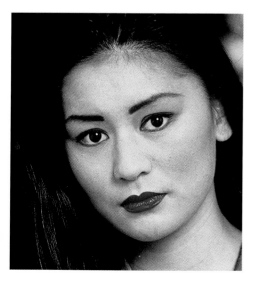

for newborns, was about to lose her job. She was missing too much time from work. Part of her job was to help parents with their grief if their baby died. But she herself felt so much grief each time a tiny patient died that, for days afterward, she couldn't come to work.

Barbara herself had undergone three abortions. The death of each premature newborn in her unit devastated her with grief. With proper counseling Barbara was finally able to deal with the source of her depression.[24]

These stories illustrate the psychological injury that can result from abortion.

"Every woman who undergoes an abortion suffers a death experience—the death of her child," says Joanne Angelo, M.D., a professor of psychiatry at Tufts University Medical School. "This is true even if those around her try to shield her from the reality of her child's prenatal life and the grim details of the abortion procedure."[25]

A woman who has an abortion usually experiences definite reactions and emotions, Dr. Angelo points out. At first she may try to deceive herself that just "a blob of tissue" or "a product of conception" was removed in the abortion. But a woman usually knows her due date—when she would have held a baby in her arms if she had not had the abortion. Before getting the abortion, she often "begins a relationship with her child, even speaking to him or her by name in her mind," says Dr. Angelo, "asking the child's forgiveness for what she is about to do."[26]

Later, perhaps even years after the abortion, many women realize how real their unborn child's life and death were. That's when they start to face their loss and grief.

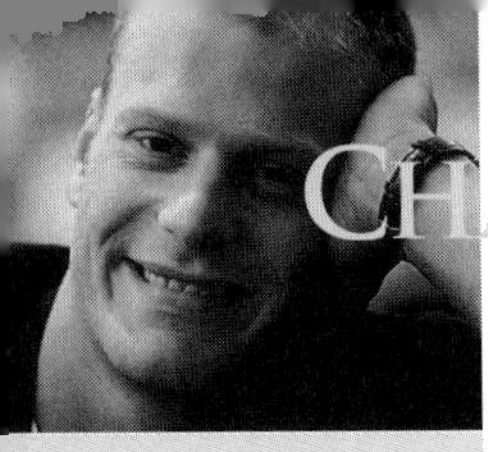

"Grief is a natural consequence of death—even prenatal death," says Dr. Angelo.[27] Many women name their aborted babies and write a letter to them as part of the healing process.

HELP FOR THE AFTERMATH

If someone you know is struggling with the emotional aftereffects of an abortion, many organizations are available to help. Pregnancy centers offer help not only for pregnant teens and women, but also for those who have had an abortion. To find a pregnancy center, a person can look in the Yellow Pages under "Abortion Alternatives" or contact the following organizations:

After Abortion Helpline
21 Violet Street
Providence, RI 02908
401-941-3050

The Elliot Institute
P.O. Box 9079
Springfield, IL 62704
217-523-2706

Institute for Pregnancy Loss
111 Bow Street
Portsmouth, NH 03801-3819
603-431-1904
Fax: 603-436-6971

National Office of Post-Abortion Reconciliation and Healing
3501 S. Lake Dr.
P.O. Box 07477
Milwaukee, WI 53207
414-483-4141
800-593-2273

Open Arms
P.O. Box 1056
Columbia, MO 65205-1056
314-449-7672
Fax: 314-442-0058

Silent Voices
191B Glover Ave.
Chula Vista, CA 91910
619-422-0757

In addition to the emotional risks, abortion also entails physical risks. These include:

- Mild to severe infection, including pelvic inflammatory disease, peritonitis, and septicemia.
- Mild to severe bleeding.
- Lacerations and perforations of the uterus, cervix, bowels, urinary tract, and other internal organs.
- Incomplete abortion or retained tissue, which can lead to bleeding and life-threatening infection.
- Infertility, as a result of scarring from the abortion itself or pelvic inflammatory disease caused by the procedure.
- Tubal pregnancy, also a result of scarring.
- Masking of a tubal/ectopic pregnancy.
- Embolism (the obstruction of a blood vessel, usually by air bubbles or blood clots).
- Complications from anesthesia and other drugs. Such complications include low blood pressure, irregular heartbeat, life-threatening fever, allergic reactions, impaired breathing, vomiting and aspiration (throwing up and then inhaling vomit), and airway obstruction.
- Disseminated intravascular coagulation (abnormal blood clotting that can lead to uncontrollable internal bleeding).
- Death.

No one really knows how often these consequences occur. The quality of the data has typically been very poor. *The Washington Times* reported one federal health official as saying, "There have always been problems identifying death secondary to abortions." Furthermore, "death certificates are not the best source of death information," the official remarked, "and we've always had concerns we're not getting all the deaths through the death certificate system."[28]

Although the federally run Centers for Disease Control keeps track of deaths due to complications of abortion, they get their data from state health departments, which differ greatly in how they collect and classify information about deaths. In addition, examiners who fill out the death certificates may not fully state the cause of death. For example, if a woman dies from an embolism caused by an abortion, the cause of death may simply be reported as an embolism rather than the abortion. The same is true for abortion deaths due to infection, hemorrhage, or anesthesia.

In one case, a North Carolina woman died of complications following an elective abortion. Although an autopsy was done, the death certificate made no mention of the abortion.[29] In another case, the death certificate of an Alabama woman categorized the cause of death as postpartum hemorrhage, which is normally a complication of labor and delivery. The coroner, however, indicated that the cause of death was "coagulation complications following abortion of a second-trimester fetus."[30]

Injuries and other complications of abortion may also be greatly underreported. Many women who are injured do not want it known that they had an abortion. Also, if they are experiencing guilt, they may feel they simply got what they deserved.

Anyone who is thinking about having an abortion needs to ask some hard questions and get some straight answers so that she can understand the risks and make the best decision possible. In particular, she has the right to know the answers to the following questions:

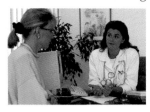

- Is the abortion center's doctor licensed to practice medicine in her state?
- Has anyone lodged complaints against the doctor with her state's medical board? Has the medical board taken any disciplinary action against the doctor?
- Has the abortion center ever been sued for injury incurred during an abortion?
- What are the possible physical and emotional side effects of the abortion procedure that will be used?
- Does the doctor have malpractice insurance that will protect her in case of a problem? Does the abortion center?
- Does the doctor have admitting privileges at a nearby hospital? If physical complications occur, will he see her in the hospital?
- Are the clinic's facilities clean? Has the equipment been adequately sterilized?
- What kind of screening takes place to avoid anesthesia complications and discover relevant preexisting conditions?
- Does the abortion clinic have the personnel and equipment to deal adequately with medical emergencies that could arise from the procedure?

If the abortion center's doctor and staff refuse to answer these questions, or try to evade them, a woman should not be afraid to walk out. She should also leave if any of the answers given raise doubts or concerns.

Besides finding out about the clinic (its personnel, equipment, and doctor), the woman needs to find out about the baby inside her. She needs to know that:

- The heart begins to beat at eighteen days.
- At eight weeks the baby has all the body parts and organs that he or she will have when born.
- The brain is functioning forty days after conception.
- At ten weeks the baby can suck his or her thumb.
- At thirteen weeks the baby can hear outside sounds, including the radio and TV.

Prevention, of course, is always the best treatment for any problem. And the best way to prevent the problems described in this chapter is to avoid pregnancy altogether by postponing sex until marriage.

That may be hard to do. It will certainly require patience, self-control, and the ability to avoid tempting or risky circumstances (we'll discuss this in chapter 7). But like many things that require effort, the payoff will be worth it.

According to the laws of the United States, all doctors who perform abortions are legally obligated to uphold minimum standards of medical care. If they fail to and thus cause a patient to suffer injury or death, they are negligent and subject to legal action.

The patient has the legal right to insist that only a licensed physician perform the abortion. She also has the right to insist that the doctor have insurance that protects and/or compensates her or her surviving relatives if she suffers injury or death as a result of an abortion.

Anyone seeking an abortion should have the doctor who will perform the abortion complete the Physician Information section of the following form. She should not let anyone—including a doctor, nurse, counselor, or clinic or hospital staff member—take this form away from her. If she needs to, she should photocopy the form. She should keep it with her at all times. It is her responsibility to protect her legal rights. Any doctor who refuses to fill out completely and sign the Physician Information section should not be permitted to perform an abortion on the patient.

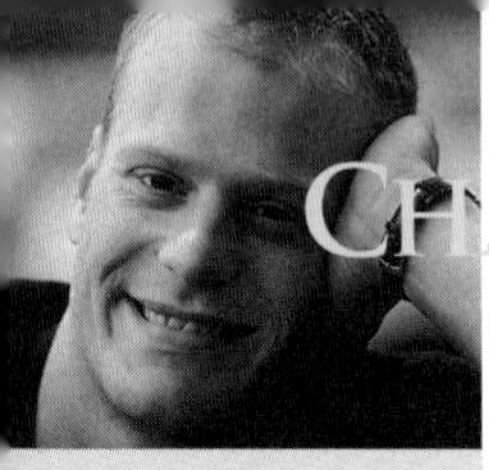

RIGHTS OF PATIENTS ABORTION DISCLOSURE FORM

Patient's name_____

Patient's address_____

_____

Telephone number_____ Date of abortion_____

Physician Information

Physician's name _____ Date of procedure _____

Facility where procedure will be performed _____

City and state of facility_____

Name of malpractice insurance company_____

City and state of malpractice insurance company _____

Policy limit $ _____ Policy number _____ Expires _____

Name of closest emergency hospital _____

Location of closest emergency hospital_____

I certify that the following is true: 1) All of the information above is true and accurate. 2) I am a physician licensed to operate in the state in which this abortion will be performed. 3) I own a malpractice insurance policy that is current and paid in full, held by the company noted on this form. 4) I do not have any unpaid or outstanding judgments or claims against me for personal injury, medical malpractice, or wrongful death. 5) If the patient named above is injured during her abortion, an ambulance will transfer her immediately to the emergency hospital noted on this form.

Physician's signature _____ Date _____

Before performing an abortion, some providers demand that their patients sign a release form stating that they will not hold the physician or clinic responsible for any harm occurring during the procedure. Such a release form carries almost no legal weight. If a patient is harmed physically or emotionally during an abortion, she always retains her legal right to seek financial compensation— *no matter what she may have signed.*

If a patient suffers harm during an abortion, but cannot afford to pay an attorney, she should still seek legal representation. Many attorneys will work with her on a contingency basis. In other words, they will not charge her a fee up front; instead they will accept a share of any settlement she might win. Another thing she should do is file a complaint with the state board of medicine.

If she has questions and wants to discuss her injury with someone, she should contact a competent medical malpractice or personal injury attorney. She might look under "Attorneys" in the Yellow Pages, call the bar association in her state capital, or contact a legal aid organization in her city or county.

There is also a growing number of organizations and attorneys who specialize in abortion malpractice. Here are some organizations an individual might contact:

American Rights Coalition
P.O. Box 487
Chattanooga, TN 37401
800-634-2224
615-624-1111

Life Dynamics
P.O. Box 2226
Denton, TX 76202
817-380-8800

Bird and Associates
1150 Monarch Plaza
3414 Peachtree Road, NE
Atlanta, GA 30326
404-264-9400

SOME HARD DECISIONS

The decision to have premarital sex may seem easy, but it often leads to some hard decisions later on.

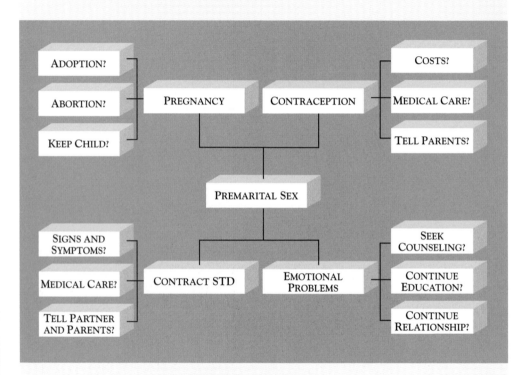

1. Who will use the contraceptive—the boy or the girl?
2. Who will pay for the contraceptives? Where will they be purchased? Will a doctor's visit be necessary?
3. Who will pay for the periodic checkups if the pill, an IUD, or a diaphragm is used?
4. What about the risks associated with contraception?
5. Will the parents of the boy and girl know about their decision?
6. What about the risk of STDs?
   • Do you know the signs and symptoms of the most common STDs?
   • If either of you contracts an STD, how will you get medical attention—health department, private doctor, etc.?

- Who will pay for medical care?
- Will the parents know if you contract an STD? What if one of you needs treatment? Will the parents be told then?
- Will the partner be told if the other one acquires an STD?
7. Because no form of contraception is 100 percent effective, what happens if the girl gets pregnant?

IF YOU CHOOSE TO ABORT...

1. Will the father know about the decision? Will he be included in the decision?
2. Will the parents of the girl know of her decision? Will the boy's parents know?
3. Where will the abortion be performed—in a clinic, at the doctor's office, or in a hospital?
4. Who will pay for the abortion—the father, the mother's family, a friend?
5. What happens if the abortion causes problems (physical or emotional)? Will the girl or boy seek counseling? Will someone sue?
6. Will the relationship continue after the abortion?

IF YOU CHOOSE TO PUT THE CHILD UP FOR ADOPTION...

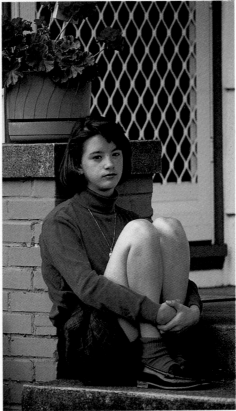

1. Will the teenage father be included in the decision-making process?
2. Will the teenagers' parents be involved in the decision-making?
3. Will the baby be placed for adoption by an agency, or will it be done privately? Will it be an open adoption or a closed adoption?
4. Who will pay for the adoption, lawyer's fees, etc.? Who will pay for prenatal care?
5. Will the baby be born in a hospital? If physical complications occur, who will be involved? What if you as the biological mother change your mind?

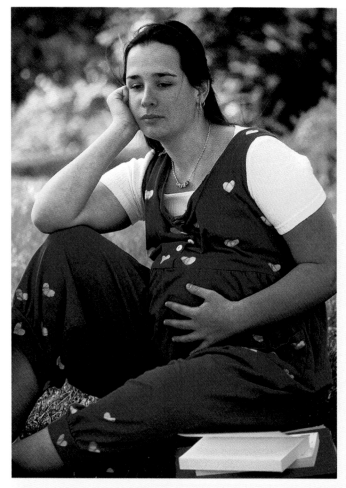

6. Will post-adoption counseling be needed? Who will pay for the counseling?

7. Will your relationship with the father continue after the adoption?

IF YOU CHOOSE TO KEEP THE CHILD...

1. Will the teenage father be part of the decision-making?
2. Will the couple get married?
3. Who will pay for the baby's needs? Will the father contribute? Will the mother get a job?
4. Will the mother's parents raise the child? Will the father's parents be involved?
5. Will the mother drop out of school? What will she do about school during her pregnancy?
6. How will the baby's health care be provided—private doctor or clinic? Who will pay for it?
7. Who will take care of the child if the mother stays in school? Who will care for the child if the mother works? Who will pay for child care?

WHICH DECISION LOOKS THE EASIEST, SAFEST, AND HEALTHIEST?

The decision to practice or regain sexual self-control looks like the most difficult one at first. But given the alternatives, saying NO to premarital sex is the best choice. The decision to be sexually active has emotional, moral, intellectual, and social consequences. Before acting, you need to consider these consequences.

1. All parents experience challenges raising their children. Why do single parents encounter so many more challenges than two parents?

2. Why is a baby almost always better off in a two-parent home?

3. How are unmarried birth mothers who choose to place their baby for adoption better off than unmarried birth mothers who keep their baby? Discuss the well-being of the children in both situations.

4. Who suffers from an abortion?

5. Abortion may seem like a simple decision, but what are some of the physical and emotional consequences of this decision?

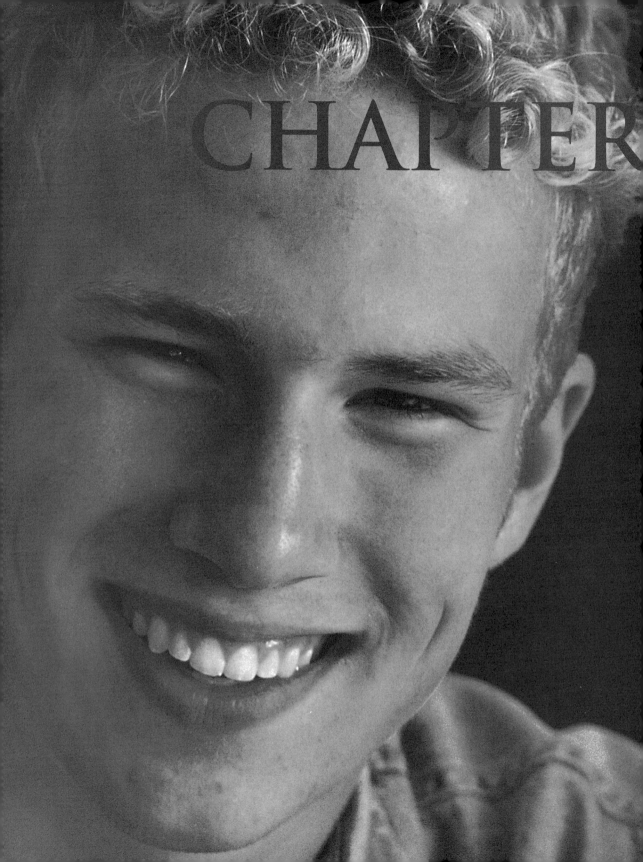

CHAPTER

6

RISKY BUSINESS: EMOTIONS

Kira Wallace, four and a half years old, plays quietly in the front yard of her grandparents' home in Coeur D'Alene, Idaho. Her mother, Shelley Parsons, and her grandmother are sitting nearby.

Kira looks up when a cream-colored pickup truck drives down the street in front of the house.

"There goes my daddy. He's coming to see me," says the little girl with pale skin, blue eyes, and wavy brown hair.

But the man in the pickup truck is not her father. Her mother and her grandmother are silent. They have nothing to say to this child who waits eagerly for her daddy to come. She's been waiting a long time.

Shelley was a junior in high school when she met nineteen-year-old Callie Wallace. He was a kind, soft-spoken young man who seemed to love children. He went fishing with Shelley's nephew and would sometimes baby-sit.

When Shelley was with Callie, she couldn't help but think of her own father. Shelley's father was a painter, but Shelley thought he was a prince. As a little girl, she'd wait for him to come home in his brown pickup truck.

"I thought he was the strongest man alive," she recalls.

After dating Callie for three months, Shelley got pregnant. They moved into his parents' home in Lowell, Oregon. Callie returned to his old friends and old habits of staying out late and coming home just in time to sleep.

Soon after their daughter's birth, Shelley moved back to her parents' home in Idaho.

She never saw Callie again. He would call, but he never visited his daughter and never sent money to support her.

"I don't need a man," Shelley decided. "Kira and I can be a family on our own."

Over the next few years Shelley worked at two jobs to support herself and her daughter in their new apartment. During that time she found out that Callie had married and started a family. She decided she had to put the past behind her and go on. She won custody of Kira and, in exchange, gave up her right to financial support.

It wasn't as easy for Kira. At the day care center, Kira saw fathers pick up their children. The little girl who was

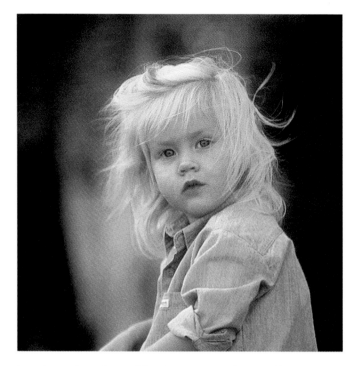

parents' home.

"I only thought about myself and Callie when I got pregnant," Shelley admits. "I assumed everything else would work out. Now I see how my decisions have hurt my daughter for the rest of her life. I feel like I cheated her out of a dad—the part of my own childhood I cherished most."[1]

Previous chapters looked at the physical consequences of premarital sex. Premarital sex also carries emotional consequences—for the child, the mother, and, though this story doesn't reveal them, the father. One consequence for Kira is an unfulfilled hunger for a father's love. For all practical purposes the little girl has no daddy. The father's absence often carries other psychological consequences for a girl, including low self-esteem, drug use, and early sexual activity (as a search for male attention and approval). The father's absence brings deep suffering to a child.

Shelley also experiences painful emotional consequences. She has to witness her daughter's longing for a father. She also suffers from the fear of commitment that often follows a broken sexual relationship. In Shelley's case, that fear is compounded by the concern that her daughter would be hurt again, perhaps even more traumatically, if a man became a seeming father-to-be—and then walked out of her life.

Shelley's reluctance to involve herself in a relationship after her daughter was

her best friend would often go to the store with her father. Kira watched them going off together one day and said, "Look! There's Stephanie and her daddy." A short time later she said she was going to buy a daddy at the store.

Then the little girl created a father. She told her mother, "My daddy has a dog," or, when Shelley asked her to clean up her room, "My daddy doesn't make me."

"If I could wish for one thing, it would be that Kira had a father," Shelley says.

But she is afraid of anything more than an occasional date. She doesn't want her little girl to get attached to a man who may not stay.

Not only does Kira not have a father, she also spends very little time with her mother since Shelley works at two jobs. Some nights she's already asleep when Shelley picks her up at her grand-

born is not unusual. Family researcher Barbara Dafoe Whitehead reports that "a significant number of all single mothers never marry or remarry. Those who do marry or remarry, do so only after spending an average of about six years as single parents."[2]

Premature sex brings with it many other emotional consequences as well, which may differ from one person to another. Some hurts may last a few days or months, while others may last for years. Some, like the consequences experienced by Shelley Parsons and her daughter, Kira Wallace, will last a lifetime. Let's look at just a few of the risks.

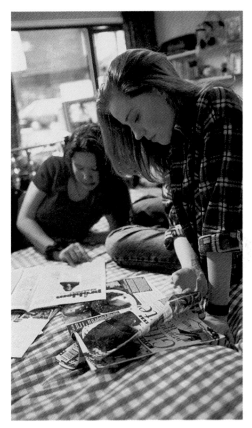

WORRY ABOUT PREGNANCY AND DISEASE

Nothing could change the way Lisa felt this morning—nothing except knowing for sure that she wasn't pregnant. Her boyfriend had talked her into sleeping with him last night. Now all she could think about was not getting pregnant. It was the first time for her, and he said it was his first time too. She told herself that at least she didn't have to worry about getting AIDS.

Not so for Lisa's best friend, Ellie. Ellie and her boyfriend, Matt, had been having sex ever since they started dating two years ago. Matt was the only person Ellie had ever had sex with. But Ellie was not the first for Matt, as she found out much later. He was infected with HIV. Now Ellie was terrified that she too would be infected.

The possibility of getting pregnant or becoming infected with a deadly sexually transmitted disease is very real. But even people who escape those consequences often fall prey to fear and anxiety.

"I see kids going to the nurses in schools, crying a day after their first sexual experience and wanting to be tested for AIDS," says Russell Henke, a health education coordinator for the Montgomery County Public Schools in Maryland. "They have done it, and now they are terrified. For some of them, that's enough. They say, 'I don't want to have to go through that experience anymore.'"[3]

"I see some of my friends buying home-pregnancy tests," a high school girl told a nurse, "and they are so worried and so distracted every month, afraid that they might be pregnant. It's a relief to me to be a virgin."[4]

REGRET AND SELF-REPROACH

Another emotional risk of premature sexual involvement is regret.

"I guess one of my biggest reasons [for becoming sexually active] was that I was curious," wrote one girl in a survey of high school and college students. "I thought and still think he loves me, and we haven't been sexually active in a month. But I can't ever get back my virginity, and that hurts."

Another teenager, eighteen years old, was less than a month from being married when her boyfriend broke off their engagement after learning she could never have children. During the years before her engagement, she had slept with several boys. Somewhere along the line she had contracted gonorrhea, but she didn't find out until a month before the wedding.

"The doctor said it will keep me

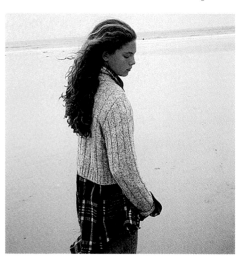

from motherhood," she said. "I wish I were dead."[5]

Regret is a common thread running through these and many other stories in this book. We see it, for example, in Tanya, who wished she could be part of a family again; in Shelley, who lives with her daughter's hurt; and in Akiko, who isolated herself each month to mourn the anniversary of her abortion.

Often the regret comes from violating one's conscience. Psychologist Henry Brandt has heard many stories from young people who have experienced heavy petting or unmarried sex. They describe their feelings this way: "First, there was great pleasure in it. Then I started hating myself. Next I found myself hating my partner. We ended up embarrassed and ashamed. Then we broke up and became enemies."[6]

Regret from violating one's conscience becomes even worse when there is manipulation. Girls are perhaps more vulnerable than boys because they are more likely to think that sex equals commitment.

In an earlier story we met Susan, who chose to have sex with her boyfriend just to fit in when she moved to a new high school. Whenever she and Greg had sex, she always felt "like a piece of trash" the next morning. But she endured the accusations of her conscience because she thought Greg loved her.

Eventually, though, Greg broke up with her.

"I wasn't expecting that at all," says Susan. "I couldn't believe it. The only person that I thought cared about me actually didn't. I felt like my whole life was nothing. I felt so used."[7]

Even though girls may be more

vulnerable to regret, boys are not immune. They, too, may regret giving in to pressure or being manipulated into violating their conscience. They may also regret actions that hurt others. In chapter 3, we saw 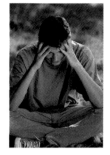 how one college student felt after dumping his girlfriend:

> *I finally got a girl into bed—actually it was in a car—when I was 17. I thought it was the hottest thing there was, but then she started saying she loved me and getting clingy....*
>
> *I was amazed to find that after four weeks of having sex as often as I wanted, I was tired of her. I didn't see any point in continuing the relationship. I finally dumped her, which made me feel even worse, because I could see that she was hurting. I felt pretty low.*[8]

Of course, that regret only becomes worse if there are also physical consequences.

GUILT AND DEPRESSION

Marsha, a twenty-eight-year-old teacher, and Bill, a young plumber, had become good friends. They had a lot in common. The more they were together, the deeper their love for one another seemed to grow.

Bill, however, said he wouldn't marry Marsha unless they found out first if they were sexually compatible. She couldn't agree with that since she believed sex was for marriage only. To "test" their compatibility, even though she loved Bill, went against all her beliefs and feelings.

But Bill insisted. He said he wouldn't marry Marsha without trying it first.

Feeling guilty and anxious, Marsha reluctantly submitted to having sex because she didn't want to lose him.

As any good marriage counselor would realize, Marsha's guilt and fear inhibited her so much that the experiment failed. This convinced Bill that he and Marsha were sexually incompatible. He broke the engagement and left his fiancée in a state of shock and depression.[9]

Guilt is closely linked to regret. We often regret our actions because of guilt. Although guilt is often perceived as a negative consequence of unmarried sex,

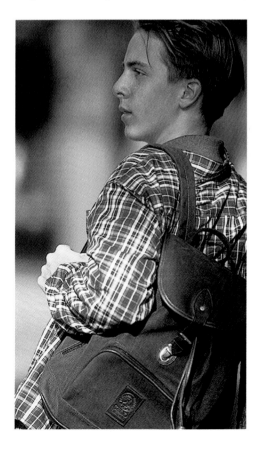

it can, however, prompt us to do the right thing and help us develop good character. One teenage boy said he stopped being sexually active when he saw how much pain he was causing the girls. "You see them crying and confused. They say they love you, but you don't love them." He said he felt guilty about that.[10]

Developmental psychologist Tom Lickona observes, "Guilt is a special form of regret—a strong sense of having done something morally wrong. Guilt is a normal and healthy moral response, a sign that one's conscience is working."[11]

Even with today's sexual freedom, if you are sexually active, you may feel guilty about what you are doing. Your conscience may bother you because you know you have hurt someone or because you know your parents would be upset if they found out you were sexually active.

But you can also feel guilty for the act itself, even if you don't think you have hurt anyone. That's not strange or odd. It simply indicates what you think deep inside. Rather than denying or dismissing that part of yourself, which can lead to emotional and even physical turmoil, you should give it a fair hearing—and then act accordingly.

Although guilt can be healthy and constructive, it can also be a lingering wound. In a college survey reported by *USA Today*, about half of the respondents said they were sorry they had engaged in premarital sex. Nearly 30 percent said they found it hard to forgive themselves.[12]

Guilt about one's sexual past may cripple people when they become parents. They may feel reluctant to advise their own children to wait for marriage. "Because these parents can't bear to be considered hypocrites, or to consider themselves hypocrites," says counselor Carson Daly, "they don't give their children the sexual guidance they very much need."[13] Yet these are the parents who should want their children not to make the same mistakes they did.

Guilt can also make people feel that they deserve any misfortune that befalls them. As we noted in the previous chapter, women who have been harmed by an abortion frequently keep silent about their injuries because they are ashamed of the abortion and think they got what they deserved.

LOSS OF SELF-RESPECT

Along with guilt and regret comes the loss of self-respect. When we violate our own standards, it's often hard to see ourselves as worthy of any respect—from either ourselves or others. What's worse, when we lose our self-respect, we damage an important barrier against further lapses, setting up a vicious cycle.

Susan, whom we discussed earlier, lost respect for herself when she started having sex with Greg. When he broke up with her, she tried to make herself feel better—boost her self-esteem—by having sex with other boys. Instead, she lost even more respect for herself.

"Joan," a college senior working as the director of a dormitory, noted a similar pattern with some of the college students in her dormitory:

There are girls in our dorm who have had multiple pregnancies and multiple abortions. They tend to be filled with self-loathing. But because they have so little self-esteem, they will settle for any kind of

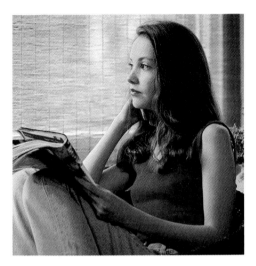

attention from guys. So they keep going back to the same kind of destructive situations and relationships that got them into trouble in the first place.[14]

Here is how one young woman who was able to pull out of this cycle describes her experience:

One thing my old boyfriend was right about was that after you do it once, it's easy to do it again. And I did, with several other guys, sometimes during a one-night stand, sometimes in long-term relationships....

One time at college, I was fooling around pretty heavily with a "stud" on campus. When I told him I didn't want to go all the way, he told me he didn't want to be friends if I wouldn't sleep with him. All of a sudden I realized what a jerk—to put it mildly—this guy was and despised myself almost as much as I did him. Needless to say, he no longer pursued me after I said no. It was a truly degrading experience then and each time I saw him around school....

Sex between two people united in love and marriage is a beautiful thing; but taken out of its proper context, sex can be destructive.

I have since put this lesson into practice and found the truth of it in my own life. After dating a guy for about a month, I broke it off and felt no self-condemnation, remorse, or embarrassment—all because I had not slept with him. And I am proud of myself!

As of yet, I haven't been in a long-term relationship, but I have no doubts it will be difficult to abstain. But if a man isn't caring or sensitive enough to respect me and my decision, I know that I don't want him in my life anyway.[15]

Casual sex can lower the self-respect of user and used alike, making real intimacy unattainable.

"You feel pretty crummy when you get drunk at a party and have sex with some girl," admitted a twenty-year-old college male, "and then the next morning you can't even remember who she was."[16]

When we treat people like things, we hurt them and lose respect for ourselves.

LOSS OF REPUTATION

Still another risk of unmarried sex is loss of reputation. Teens who become sexually active one day may find their reputations gone the next. Other teens may hold them in contempt, gossip and joke about them behind their backs, say cruel things to them directly, or shun them.

For girls it may also mean that boys ask them out in hopes of "scoring," as the following letter to Ann Landers illustrates.

The letter from "Fourth Choice" hit home. The anti-make-outs were unhappy because they had no dates. They said the

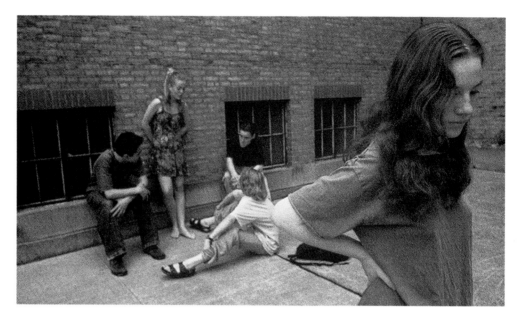

fast girls were rushed to death. Well, Ann, I'm one of the fast girls, and I'd like to tell you how it looks from here.

I get asked out every night of the week, and I'm sick of these creeps who want to make out all the time. I am also sick of myself. I'm only 17, and my reputation isn't worth [a nickel]. My girlfriends tell me what they hear about me from their brothers, and of course I deny everything. I know now that nine guys out of ten can't be trusted to keep their mouths shut. Whenever I meet a new [guy] I wonder how much he has heard.

Please tell "Fourth Choice" that I wish I could change places with her.[17]

Sadly, this girl is making another mistake if she thinks it's too late to save her reputation. In fact, she can make a fresh start and regain the advantages of an abstinent lifestyle. She can choose secondary virginity and practice sexual self-control until she marries. Also, she can let her friends—and the boys she dates—know she has made that deci-

sion. The word will get around fast.

REDUCED ABILITY TO TRUST AND FEAR OF COMMITMENT

Teens and adults who feel betrayed or cheapened after a sexual relationship may find it difficult to trust others or commit themselves in future relationships. This is another risk of unmarried sex. As we saw in the previous letter to Ann Landers, girls may be suspicious when boys seek them out. Likewise boys may become suspicious when girls show interest, afraid they'll get burned again.

Although some, like Susan, lose their self-esteem and go from relationship to relationship, many others withdraw. We saw this with Shelley Parsons, whom we discussed at the beginning of this chapter. After Callie Wallace, the father of her child, lost interest and married someone else, Shelley was afraid to get involved again. She dated only occasionally because she didn't want her daughter, Kira, to become attached to a man who might not stay around, and because she herself had come to fear attachment.

Girls are usually the ones who get hurt and pull back from trusting. They think boys are out only for sex. As one young woman put it, "Besides feeling cheap [after several sexual relationships], I began to wonder if there would ever be anyone who would love and accept me without demanding that I do something with my body to earn that love."[18]

Boys, however, can also lose their ability to trust girls, fearing to make a commitment after a sexual relationship ends. One college student tells his experience:

I first had intercourse with my girl-friend when we were fifteen. I'd been going with her for almost a year, and I loved her very much. She was friendly and outgoing. We'd done every-thing but have intercourse, and then one night she asked if we could go all the way.

A few days later, we broke up. It was the most painful time of my life. I had opened myself up to her more than I had to anybody, even my parents.

I was depressed, moody, nervous. My friends dropped me because I was so bummed out. I felt like a failure. I dropped out of sports. My grades weren't terrific.

I didn't go out again until I got to college. I've had

mostly one-night stands in the last couple of years.

I'm afraid of falling in love.[19]

Another risk of unmarried sex comes when sexually active teens become so absorbed in a sexual relationship that they neglect other aspects of their lives. At the very time when they should be finding new friends, joining sports teams or service clubs, developing their abilities and hobbies, and taking on civic responsibilities, they find themselves expending all their energy on a sexual relationship and all that it brings.

That's what happened to Jennifer Stratton and Randy Parker. Before sex entered the picture, they were active at

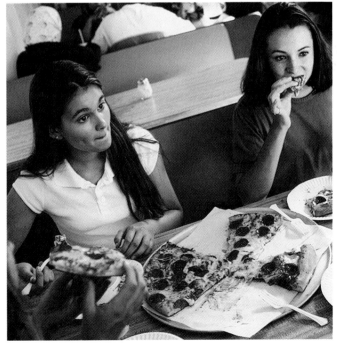

school and looking forward to college. But once sex became the focus, they argued a lot and lost interest in school activities, family get-togethers, and college. By giving in to Randy, Jennifer not only saw her relationship with Randy disintegrate, but she also missed experiences important for her personal development and her future.

Outside interests are "important nutrients for a teenager's development as a person," says psychologist Tom Lickona. "And this period of life is special because young people have both the time and the opportunities to develop their talents and interests. The growing they do during these years will affect them all their lives. If young people don't put these years to good use, they may never develop their full potential."[20]

Sexually active girls seem to be at greater risk for letting this happen. According to New York psychiatrist Samuel Kaufman, "A girl who enters into a serious relationship with a boy very early in life may find out later that her individuality was thwarted. She became part of him and failed to develop her own interests, her sense of independent identity."[21]

RAGE OVER BETRAYAL

After a sexual relationship breaks up, the partner who was dumped may become enraged. This is another serious emotional risk of unmarried sex. Consider the countless acts of violence against former girlfriends or boyfriends by jilted lovers. Sex is almost always a major player here.

You may feel angry if your boyfriend

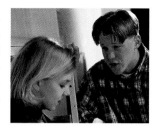

or girlfriend breaks up with you, but the feelings run deeper if you have engaged in sexual intimacy.

"Sex can be emotional dynamite," says Tom Lickona. "It can lead a person to think that the relationship is really serious, that both people really love each other. It can create a very strong emotional bond that hurts terribly when it's ruptured—especially if it seems that the other person never had the same commitment. And the resulting sense of betrayal can give rise to rage, even violence."[22]

As one teen said, "You get hurt every time you have sex, then break up—the emotional pain doesn't go away."[23]

NEGATIVE EFFECTS ON SEXUAL INTIMACY IN MARRIAGE

Sex before marriage can put you at risk for having serious sexual problems after marriage. You may have such a bad experience with sex that you get turned off by it. Later, after getting married, it may be difficult for you to enjoy this beautiful part of marriage.

You may even compare your mate with former sex partners, basing your comparison on someone else's performance. And, of course, your partner might do the same to you.

Flashbacks of premarital sexual experiences can also intrude when you and your mate are enjoying sexual intimacy. You may not realize it at the time, but sexual encounters before marriage can be stored in your mind, only to appear and remind you of the past.

Jean, a young woman in her thirties, visited a psychologist because of marital problems. Her husband was the man of her dreams. Their two children gave them great joy. But Jean was so disturbed by flashbacks that she sought counseling.

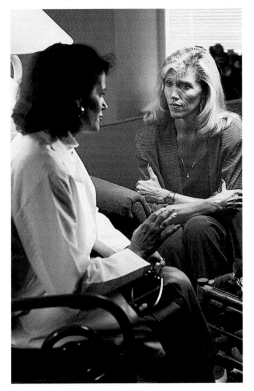

"When Michael and I make love and I look into his eyes and feel his arms around me, I suddenly see Jack...or Ron ...or Steve," she told the psychologist. "I didn't even like Steve. It was a terrible relationship. But the thought of these men is ruining my desire for my husband. And now Michael and I are having awful problems with sex in our marriage."[24]

Incidentally, even if you've never had sex, you can develop similar problems if you use pornography. Researchers at the University of Alabama at Birmingham have found that people exposed to pornography reported diminished satisfaction with their partner's physical appearance, affection, curiosity, and performance. The researchers warned that such dissatisfaction could "instigate many men and women to seek out conditions that promise more and better sexually gratifying experiences."[25]

SPIRITUAL IMPLICATIONS

So far we have considered the moral, physical, and emotional aspects of sex. But sex also has a spiritual aspect, which, for most people, means belief in God. Religion has always played an important role in American society.[26] Moreover, the percentage of people in America who profess belief in God has consistently been one of the highest for any country in the world. So has the percentage of people who say that their religious beliefs are very important to them.[27] With that in mind it's natural to consider the spiritual dimension of a person's sexuality.

Many faith traditions prohibit unmarried sex. In fact, the major world religions such as Judaism, Islam, and Christianity agree that unmarried sex is wrong, as is sex between two people who are married to other persons.

Young people who accept these teachings and yet engage in sex outside of marriage will most likely find that they have violated their conscience. Their actions may undermine their participation in the faith traditions to which they belong. The spiritual consequences of premarital sex can include feeling alienated from God, finding it hard to pray, falling away from practicing their faith, and losing their belief in God.

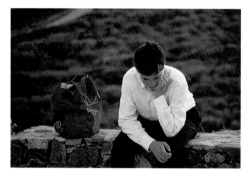

Carson Daly has counseled college students and others for many years concerning sexual matters. "I don't think I ever met a student who was sorry he or she had postponed sexual activity," she says, "but I certainly met many who deeply regretted their sexual involvements. Time and time again I have seen the long-term emotional and spiritual desolation that results from sexual promiscuity: the lowered self-esteem; the despairing sense of having been used; the self-contempt for being a user; the embarrassment of having a reputation that puts you outside the circle of people with true integrity; the unease about having to lie or at least having to conceal one's activities from family members and others; the extreme difficulty of breaking the vicious cycle of compulsive sexual behavior; and the self-hatred of seeking, after each break-up, someone else to seduce in order to revive one's fading self-image.

"No one tells students that it sometimes takes years to recover from the effects of these sexual involvements—if one ever fully recovers."[28]

Sex can provide joy and pleasure, as well as deep hurts and suffering. When enjoyed in a safe environment—one that is both physically and emotionally safe—sex is at its best and most fulfilling. Through the ages the only truly safe place for sex has been in a loving marriage. In the next chapter we'll consider how character affects your dating relationships and helps prepare you for a relationship that will last a lifetime.

1. Three things may attract you to someone of the opposite sex: some-one who's different; someone who's a challenge; and someone whom you can respect. Once you become sexually active, do you still find your partner *different*, a *challenge*, or *worthy of respect*? Discuss the relation between attraction and sexual activity.

2. Why are girls more likely to think that sex equals commitment in a relationship?

3. Psychologist Antonia Abbey has found that males have more difficulty than females distinguishing friendliness from sexual attraction.[29] Why do you think men are more likely than women to assume that friendliness implies a sexual invitation?

4. If both men and women suffer from the emotional consequences of premarital sex, why don't we hear more about how men are feeling?

5. How can comparing your spouse with former sex partners *hurt* a marriage?

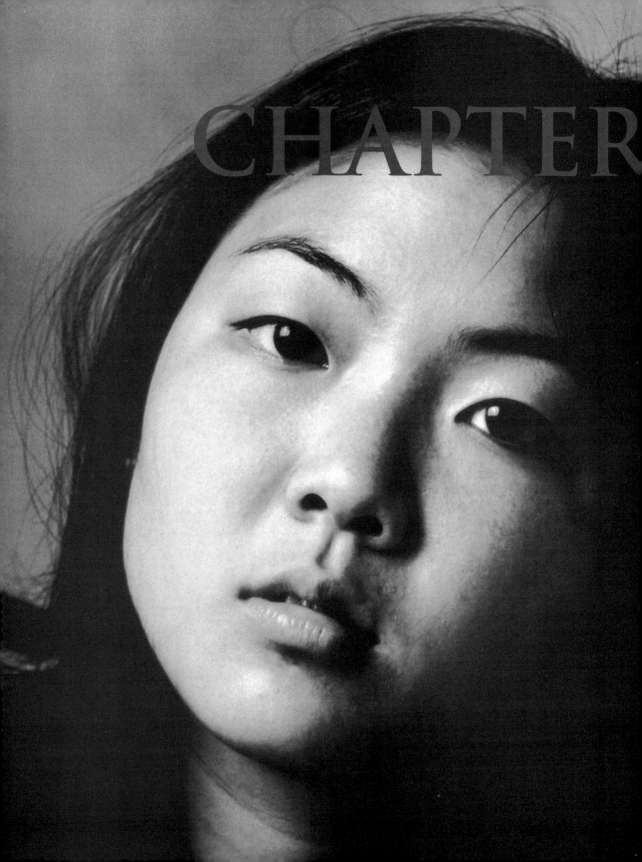

CHAPTER

7

Part of being a loving person is really caring enough about yourself and the other person to say no to things that are wrong.

CHARACTER AND DATING

-Mike and Rita Marker, from NO Is a Love Word

Dating says a lot about your character. That doesn't mean everything you do on a date has moral implications. But dating will require you to make decisions that display either good or bad character. The purpose of this chapter is to show you some of the ways character can affect your dates, help you evaluate and improve your own character in this area, and show you how to make dating more fun.

In chapter 2, we looked at the components of good character: moral knowing, moral feeling, and moral action. These components can help you understand what it means to exhibit good character on a date.

DATING AND MORAL KNOWING

SELF-KNOWLEDGE

As we noted in chapter 2, a key element of moral knowing is *self-knowledge*, or the ability to understand your own thoughts and behavior. Self-knowledge includes understanding your motives and intentions, being aware of your expectations and limitations, and being able to evaluate your actions.

Understanding your motives and intentions. An important part of evaluating

and improving your character in dating is being candid with yourself about why you want to date.

Consider Rob, for instance. Rob was known for taking his responsibilities at school and home seriously. For example, in high school he had been president of his senior class and coach of his little brother's softball team. Now that he was a freshman in college, he was making plans for his future. Rob wanted to find a wife. He knew that dating was the best way for him to find the right person. Dating would help him get to know himself better, as well as other people.

As this example illustrates, many reasons for dating are healthy and legitimate. These include:

- having fun
- getting to know someone
- developing interpersonal skills
- strengthening a relationship
- selecting a future spouse

Other reasons for dating, however, are not legitimate. These include:

- peer pressure
- being seen with someone who's popular or attractive
- making someone else jealous
- fear of not finding a future spouse
- having sex
- adding a "notch" to your belt

Try the "Front Page Test" to find out when a reason for dating is legitimate and when it isn't: How would you feel if your local newspaper published your reasons for dating on the front page? If you'd feel like a creep, you're probably dating for the wrong reasons.

Being aware of your expectations. You should also be aware of what you expect to happen on a date and whether your expectations are realistic or legitimate.

For boys, an illegitimate expectation would be expecting your date to have sex or become physically intimate with you because you've spent money on her. For both sexes, an unrealistic expectation would be expecting your date to fall in love with you the first time you go out—or even on subsequent outings. It would also be unrealistic to assume that after one or two dates you have some kind of "claim" on the other person, as if you were going steady.

Being aware of your limitations. Another important part of evaluating and improving your character is knowing your limitations on self-control and your ability to compensate for them. You need to know what kinds of activities or situations put you at risk for having sex.

For example, being at home alone with your date makes it much harder to resist the temptation to become sexually intimate. Likewise, alcohol and drugs can impair your judgment and lower

your inhibitions, causing you to do things you wouldn't normally do.

Certain social settings can also set you up for trouble. If you go to a party where people are using alcohol and drugs, or are slipping off to have sex, you are subjecting yourself to both temptation and social pressure—a combination most people find hard to resist. If you attend such parties often, your odds of giving in are even greater.

Do you remember reading about Jennifer and Randy in chapter 3? They had decided to wait until marriage to have sex, mainly because of Jennifer's desire to do so. But on the night of their prom, at a party where other couples had disappeared to the bedrooms or into the woods surrounding the house, Jennifer and Randy were left alone watching television. After some time the couple overstepped their limits, and Jennifer gave in to Randy's pleas to have sex. She regretted her choice and what it did to their relationship.

Sexual feelings become more intense as you become more intimate physically. The further you go, the less likely you are to stop.

For most people being together, holding hands, and giving each other a simple goodnight kiss may arouse romantic feelings, but not necessarily genital feelings. In general, males experience sexual arousal more quickly than females. For both sexes a good guideline is to limit physical affection to light hugs and kisses. Going further than that puts sexual feelings in the driver's seat and makes it harder to stay in control.

Being aware of warning signs. Not only do you need to know what situations to avoid, but you also need to determine when your feelings and actions are putting you in danger.

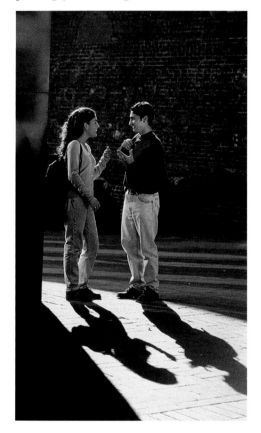

Missy's story illustrates how important this is. At the beginning of the school year Missy met Rick, a new boy in her Spanish class. They became instant friends, talking about everything that came up at school and at home. They also lived in the same neighborhood. After a few weeks their friendship deepened into a romance, and they started dating.

As Missy put it, "One thing led to another. I often wondered how far was too far, but I had decided I could stop whenever I wanted to."

When Missy went over to Rick's house, they would go to his room to be alone. It was the only place the couple could talk since Rick had a large family.

"We innocently would sit on his bed," Missy said. "After we started dating it was harder to just sit there with each other. Kissing came first, and we found it harder and harder to stop there. Even after we became involved in heavy petting, I still believed I could stop before we actually did it."

But after several months of heavy petting Missy found that she didn't want to stop. Finally, one night, she and Rick had sex.

Later, Rick walked Missy to her car and asked her what was wrong. She burst into tears.

"I hated it!" she told him. "I never want to do it again."

"I love you," Rick said.

But Missy couldn't tell him she loved him. She no longer had feelings for him. They sat in front of Rick's house for a long time and cried. They knew that what they had done together was wrong.

After that, Rick had to leave town for three weeks. While he was away, Missy thought a lot about their relationship and how it was the opposite of the way she knew a relationship should be. She realized what was right and reevaluated her moral choices. She still cared for Rick, but she knew if they were to have a relationship, they would both have to respect her deepest moral beliefs.

"Now I know that 'too far' doesn't mean only intercourse, but also the stages leading up to it," Missy said. "Too far is when you crave the physical more than anything else. Too far is when sexual thoughts take over your relationship. Too far is when you don't want to stop. It can be different for different people. It can be holding hands, kissing, or hugging. For me kissing is the limit. I've decided not to go any further than this until I'm married—and to be pure from this day on."[1]

You need to know when your feelings and actions are putting you in danger. Here are some warning signs to keep in mind. You are going too far when

- your hands or your partner's hands start to roam
- either of you starts to remove clothing
- you create in someone a desire you can fulfill only by violating moral standards
- you arouse genital feelings, or your genital feelings are aroused
- you are doing something you would not want to do around someone you really respect
- you cannot make an intelligent decision about what you should or shouldn't do
- you have doubts about whether you are doing the right thing

Another thing to watch for is your desire for acceptance. For instance, you may want others to accept you, but you don't think they do. As a result, you may feel insecure, which makes you more vulnerable to manipulation or coercion. Under such conditions you may be tempted to give in to your dating partner's demands for physical intimacy because 1) you think you will please your partner by doing so and 2) you believe physical intimacy is a sign that your partner has accepted you.

Although you may please your dating partner at first, you will probably lose your partner's respect in the long run—not to mention your self-respect. In fact, the very act that you hope will win your

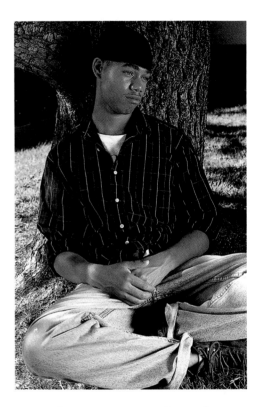

partner's respect communicates that you don't think very highly of yourself and are willing to sacrifice almost anything to be accepted.

Furthermore, you may think that physical intimacy is a sign of acceptance, love, and commitment, but your partner may not. As we saw in chapter 6, people have been badly hurt by confusing sex with acceptance, love, and commitment.

A person's self-worth can often be traced back to childhood. Parents and care providers affect a child's self-worth by the value they place on a child's gifts, talents, and efforts. Poor self-worth typically comes from a sense of inadequacy and unworthiness originating in childhood. If children receive little attention, lots of criticism, or no feedback, or if they are ignored, they may develop poor self-esteem and grow up as adults who struggle with deep feelings of inadequacy.

One reason young adults with poor self-esteem join gangs is because gangs accept their members as part of a family. Gangs typically support rather than criticize their members, and set expectations that aren't too high. Gangs accept their members unconditionally. Unfortunately, gangs also participate in violent and illegal acts. It is therefore never morally right to join a gang.

During adolescence it is normal to experience feelings of inadequacy or disappointment occasionally. Low self-worth becomes a problem, however, when it takes over your life. The following "people" have a serious problem with low self-worth:

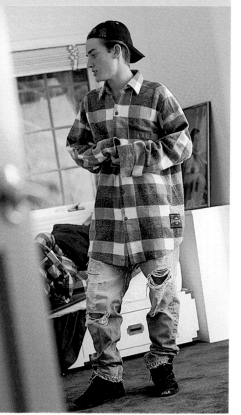

1. **Patrick Pride** deals with his poor self-image by puffing himself up. He comes across as thinking he is better than others, stuck up. You can tell Patrick from afar by the way he walks—he saunters, with his nose up in the air.

Patrick is cool and cocky. He intimidates others because he seems so sure of himself. Patrick is covering up his real feelings of insecurity. He makes up for his insecurity by cutting others down. He waits for people to say dumb or embarrassing things so he can make fun of them. He tries to make himself look good; this gives him a sense of power or control. We all know people like this—maybe one of them is even looking at you in the mirror.

Patrick and those like him may take drugs or alcohol, or engage in premarital sex, because they think these unhealthy behaviors will make them look good.

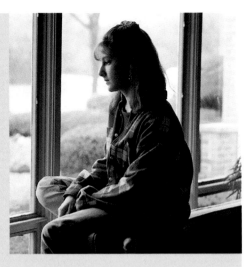

2. **Pitiful Pam** deals with not liking herself in just the opposite way from Patrick. Instead of bragging about herself, Pam puts herself down. She says things like "Oh, I'm so dumb. I can't do anything right." She knows, however, that you won't agree with her. She is counting on you to say she is wrong. Pitiful Pam is fishing for compliments.

Pam needs approval to feel good about herself. She depends on others' comments to feel good. You often find her comparing herself to others. "I wish I was as smart as Diane." "Stacy is so pretty, and I am so ugly."

Pitiful Pam is easily influenced by negative peer pressure. Because of her need to feel accepted, she is at great risk of engaging in premarital sex. But once the relationship ends—which it almost always does—she feels more unworthy and inadequate than she did before. For Pam, sex and feelings of low self-worth form a vicious cycle.

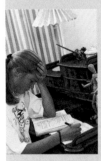

3. **Perfect Patty** pushes herself. Patty lives with unreachable expectations. She tries to achieve in music, athletics, and academics, but her workload is unrealistic. She actually sets herself up for failure.

When she is older, she will probably become a workaholic. She is overly critical and never satisfied with anything she does. In school her projects and homework are never good enough. If she does not get straight A's or come in first, she is devastated.

Patty probably isn't getting enough attention at home, except for a lot of criticism and a push for perfection. She may engage in unhealthy and inappropriate behaviors to escape the unreachable expectations demanded at home.

4. **Painful Paul** also pushes himself. He feels as if everything that goes wrong in life is his fault. He may punish himself by abusing alcohol and drugs, or if he's really seeking attention, he may resort to violence. He does not eat right, gets little sleep, and does not exercise.

You can recognize Paul from his body language. You rarely see his eyes. He seems to hate everyone. He drives too fast and is reckless.

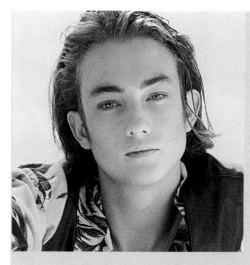

Paul easily gets involved in dangerous behaviors, like taking drugs or alcohol, because he cares little about himself. It may also be because he cares little about others. He doesn't think about the future consequences of his behavior.

All four of these people have developed low self-worth. Low self-worth can change. We all experience times when we don't feel good about ourselves. But those feelings come and go. The way to improve our self-worth and gain self-esteem is by developing our character.

It may surprise you that many people who seem confident on the outside actually feel miserable on the inside. People with low self-worth often focus too much on themselves. Thinking of others is a good way to improve low self-worth. Focusing on others is also a good way to overcome depression—it helps to realize that there are always people worse off than you.

SIX KEYS TO A HEALTHY RELATIONSHIP

1. **Communication**: Clear expression of thoughts and feelings both verbally and nonverbally. For example, being a good listener.

2. **Commitment**: Sticking to your promises and agreements; loyalty; reliability; being faithful through good times and bad. For example, completing assignments.

3. **Self-Control**: Ability to control feelings; speaking and acting calmly even though you may be angry; doing what is right without

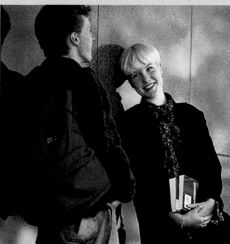

individuals having to watch you. For example, avoiding drugs, alcohol, and pornography.

4. **Compatibility**: Working together in harmony; having similar goals and aspirations; enjoying the same things; not simply using the same things or occupying the same space. For example, celebrating birthdays with siblings.

5. **Trustworthiness**: Earning people's trust; they can count on you; you keep your word even though you may not feel like it. For example, fulfilling family responsibilities.

6. **Love**: A daily decision to look out for the other person not solely based on feelings; to care for someone deeply even though your feelings may not be returned; sacrifice. For example, taking the time to visit a friend in the hospital.

KNOWLEDGE OF MORAL VALUES

Another element of moral knowing is understanding what moral values are relevant to dating—and understanding how to apply them. Two important values are respect and responsibility.

Respect. As we saw in chapter 2, respect means recognizing someone's worth and treating that person accordingly. You can demonstrate respect on a date in many ways. For example,

- Ask the person out in advance, instead of at the last minute. Asking in advance is considerate and communicates that both the person and the outing are important to you.
- Dress appropriately. Make sure your clothes fit the occasion and won't embarrass or insult your date. Never wear revealing or seductive clothes.
- Be courteous and considerate. Boys: pick up your date at the door, instead of sitting in the car and honking the horn.

- Introduce your date to your parents.
- Talk to and show interest in your date's parents if you are the one being introduced.
- While on your date, don't talk about the cost of the date or about past relationships.
- Don't engage in reckless behavior that could harm, frighten, or embarrass your date.
- Don't ignore your date or spend much of your time talking to everybody else.

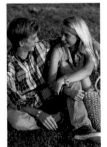

- Show gratitude for your date's courtesy and company. (Don't wait until the outing is over to say thank you.)
- Pay attention to your date while the two of you are talking.
- Maintain good eye contact to show you're really listening.
- Give feedback by nodding your head

occasionally and saying yes, unless you disagree.

- Ask questions if you don't understand exactly what your date is saying. Or summarize briefly what you thought your date said, just to make sure you heard correctly.
- Try to take your date's point of view and imagine how he or she might be feeling.
- Do not make sexual advances or pressure your date for sex—no matter how much money has been spent on the outing.

Responsibility. Responsibility is an extension of respect. It includes looking out for the good of your dating partner. It also includes being dependable and trustworthy. You show responsibility when you:

- Plan your outing.
- Determine the cost ahead of time and decide who will pay for what.
- Meet your date on time.
- Tell your parents whom you're going out with, what the person is like, where you are going, and when you'll be home.
- Get home on time.

PERSPECTIVE-TAKING

One of the keys to interacting successfully with anyone is taking the other person's point of view. In dating this means anticipating what your partner might think about your words, actions, or appearance. Taking another person's point of view is an important part of demonstrating respect and responsibility. Are you using words or expressions that your partner might find offensive or embarrassing? Are you talking about topics that make your

partner uncomfortable? Are your clothing and behavior encouraging the wrong expectations? Asking yourself these kinds of questions—and answering them realistically—can mean the difference between a good date and a bad one.

Think about your date's future. Remember that you are dating someone's future husband or wife. How would you like your future husband or wife to be treated right now? For example, would you want your future spouse to be gaining as much sexual experience as he or she could, with someone else, prior to marrying you?

DATING AND MORAL INTEGRITY

CONSCIENCE

As was mentioned in chapter 2, a healthy conscience helps us resist temptation by making us feel guilty when we do something wrong. Ideally, our conscience stops us before we do something wrong. But sometimes it needs help. As temptation and desire become more intense, it's often easy to silence our conscience temporarily by rationalizing what we want to do. For example, to justify having sex, we might say things like:

- "We're using protection, so no one will get hurt."
- "It's OK because we really love each other."
- "This is the only way to find out if we're compatible."
- "What I'm doing is right because it makes him happy."
- "This is what people our age are supposed to do."

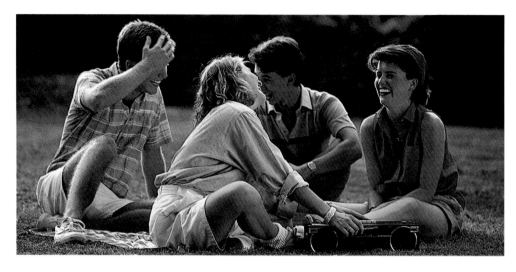

We can give our conscience some badly needed help by taking advantage of the human tendency to behave well when others are looking. Quite often, our conscience seems to work better when other people are looking on or when we know that others will find out what we've done. We can take advantage of that tendency in two ways.

One way is to make sure you and your date remain in the presence of others. This may mean going out with other couples or going places where there's not enough privacy for anything more than quiet talk or a simple kiss.

Another way, if you can't stay in the presence of others, is to make yourself accountable to others. You can do that by ensuring that someone else always finds out what you did on your date. To make yourself accountable, you will need to do three things:

First, set clear standards ahead of time. Such standards include:

- "I will keep myself pure for the person I marry."
- "I will not pet."
- "I will not be alone with my date in my house or my date's."
- "I will not use alcohol or drugs."
- "I will not go to parties where people are drinking, taking drugs, or having sex."

Second, communicate those standards to a trusted friend, family member, or mentor who agrees with what you're trying to do and who is willing to hold you to your commitment. You should also communicate your standards to your date at the very beginning of your outing. (Be aware, however, that people are sometimes tempted by what they cannot have and that your date may perceive your standards as a challenge. For instance, a girl who meets resistance from her boyfriend may try to arouse him to the point where he stops resisting and yields to her sexual advances.)

Third, after the date, tell your friend how you did. Of course, this works only if you're honest with the person you've asked to help you and if that person is willing to hold you to your standards. But doing this can give your conscience the edge you need to stay ahead of temptation.

SELF-CONTROL

To get along with other people, we all need self-control. If you always did exactly what you wanted to do or said exactly what you thought, you probably wouldn't have any friends. You might even end up in prison—or dead.

Successful dating requires self-control. What does self-control look like on a date? Self-control may mean resisting the urge to talk about yourself the whole time rather than listening to your friend. It may mean keeping your ego under control when you want to show off. Or taming a sharp tongue. Or staying cool when things don't go the way you planned. Or not pressuring your friend to go places he or she doesn't want to go.

Self-control on a date may also mean resisting the desire to have sex or become too intimate physically. As we've seen, one of the keys to self-control is a healthy conscience. Two other keys, which work together, are anticipation and avoidance.

Anticipation means knowing your limitations and weaknesses, as well as the types of situations that are likely to get you in trouble. Avoidance means staying clear of situations where you might be tempted to abandon your moral standards. This is easiest to do when you plan what you will do ahead of time (taking into account your moral standards) and stick to your plans.

If you do get into a situation where you start getting aroused or feel pressured by either your date or your peers, get out immediately. The longer you wait, the harder it will be to resist temptation or say *no* to pressure. And never make important decisions—other than to get out—in these kinds of circumstances.

EMPATHY

Put yourself in the other person's shoes. How would you feel if your date ignored you and spent the whole time talking to someone else? Or if your date tried to pressure you into doing something you didn't want to do? How would you feel if your date got you to violate your conscience?

You can also empathize better if you observe your dating partner and really listen to what he or she is saying. The more you do this, the easier it will be to treat your date with respect and care.

HUMILITY

Like self-control and empathy, humility is vital to good character—especially on a date. How much fun is it to date people who are stuck up or who keep talking about how great they are?

Humility helps you see others as being just as important as yourself. That doesn't mean you become a doormat, always giving in to other people. But it also doesn't mean treating others as doormats. A healthy sense of humility makes it easier to find a good balance.

COMPETENCE, WILL, AND HABIT

The tips and suggestions on the preceding pages will help you acquire the skills you need for exercising good character on your dates. But to use these skills, you will need one more thing: will. Will is the moral energy to put these skills into practice.

The will to do what's right is not something that just happens to you, but something you have to make happen. This may not be easy, but you can make it easier if you make it a point to exercise good character in every area of your life: in school, on the athletic field, at home, at church, with your friends, even alone in your room. The more you exercise good character and the more you make a habit of doing what you know is right, the easier it will be to keep doing the right thing when the pressure is on.

GOING STEADY AND GETTING ENGAGED

Going on a date doesn't mean you're going to go steady with your partner or get engaged, but that's how such relationships usually start. A dating relationship (as long as you don't break up) passes through several stages:

- Casual dating
- Serious dating or going steady
- Engagement
- Marriage

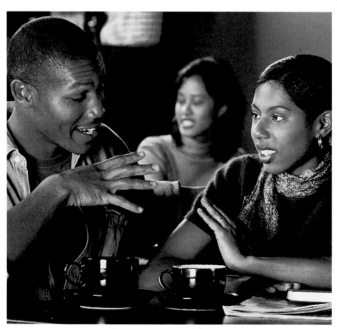

Casual dating gives you an opportunity to get to know the other person and decide what each of you likes or dislikes about the other. As the relationship matures, you may decide to go steady, that is, to date each other exclusively. As you get to know each other even better, you may decide that you're ready to make a lifelong commitment to each other. This usually means getting engaged and ultimately married.

Going steady offers several benefits:
- You can usually count on having a date for an event or activity.
- You know you have a special friend.
- You don't have to wait for the phone to ring.
- You don't have to face rejection.
- You don't have to battle the competition.

But steady relationships also carry certain risks. How you respond to those risks not only demonstrates your character, but also makes the difference between a relationship that builds you both up or tears you both down. Some of those risks are as follows:
- You may take each other for granted.
- One partner may become "clingy."
- You may spend too much time together.
- You are more likely to have sex.

Let's look at these risks one by one.

One of the dangers in any serious relationship is that people can start to take each other for granted. Once a relationship seems to be going smoothly, one or both partners may not put as much effort into the relationship as they once did. They may neglect each other or become less considerate.

For example, after a few months of steady dating, a boy may start waiting until the last minute to ask his girlfriend out. When he arrives at her house, he may honk the horn instead of going to the door. Or, once inside the house, he may ignore her family members or speak abruptly to them.

So, too, a girl may decide to go shopping with her friends instead of meeting her boyfriend for a study date at the library—without telling him so he can make other arrangements. Or, after hearing him tell the same joke several times, she may look bored the next time or remark to him in front of others that she's tired of hearing it. One partner may stop listening attentively to what the other person is saying, even cutting the other off in conversation.

If you find disrespect or irresponsibility becoming a problem in your relationship, you might try looking at things from the other person's perspective. Perhaps one of you has experienced a family crisis or illness, and hasn't been able to put the same energy into the relationship as before the crisis. You might need to show empathy to that partner and lay aside some of your own needs until the crisis passes. Or you may need to tell your partner how you've been feeling. A simple reminder can be enough to get someone back on the right track of treating others with respect and responsibility.

If you have been disrespectful or irresponsible toward your partner, you may need to look at the reasons why, talk about them if necessary with your partner or a trusted friend, and resolve to exercise self-control.

Many people, at one time or another, feel insecure about themselves or their relationships. Their self-image may be so low that they wonder how anyone could like them, let alone become involved in a romantic relationship with them. When they feel this way, it's easy for them to imag- 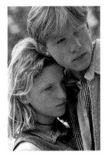 ine that their partner has lost interest in them and to interpret their partner's words and behaviors pessimistically.

When this happens, it's easy for the insecure partner to become "clingy" and want to be around the other person all the time. The insecure partner may also become jealous or demanding. This kind of behavior can start a vicious cycle: When one partner becomes clingy, the other reacts by pulling away. This only heightens the first partner's insecurity, creating even more clinging—which in turn drives the other person even farther away.

Or one partner may take advantage of the other person's low self-image by making sexual advances. But this, too, can lead to a vicious cycle. Giving in to sex often lowers the insecure partner's self-respect, making him or her even more vulnerable to the other's sexual advances.

If your partner is acting clingy, you

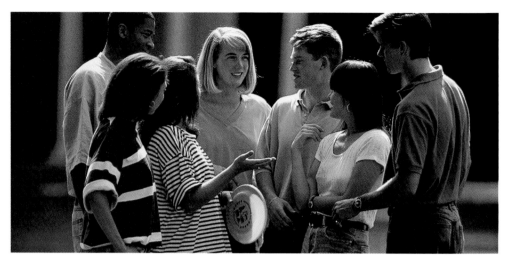

probably need to talk about it. Finding out why your partner feels insecure may help you understand why he or she interprets your words and behaviors pessimistically. It may help you be more sensitive to behaviors that trigger your partner's insecurity and prompt you to be more reassuring in situations where your partner feels insecure.

If you are the one who is clingy, you need to ask yourself if you are assessing your partner's behavior realistically. Talking to a friend may help you get a better perspective on your partner and on your relationship. If it turns out you are right in thinking that your partner is losing interest in you, pull back. That will either make you more attractive, or help to end a relationship that isn't meant to be. Either way, your dignity will be intact.

Also, getting involved in a project or hobby, especially in a group, can take your focus off each other and help you develop more confidence. Above all, never use sex to win your partner's approval or manipulate your partner into greater commitment.

SPENDING TOO MUCH TIME TOGETHER

Another risk is that a couple may spend too much time together. This may not seem like a big deal. After all, couples are supposed to spend time together. It's not the time you spend together, however, that's the problem, so much as the time you spend away from other important things.

For one thing, you may spend so much time with your partner that you neglect your friends. Most of your friends expect you to spend time with your partner. But just like anyone else they need to be treated with respect, and they need to know that you still value their friendship. No one wants to feel discarded.

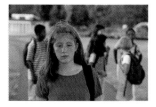

Quite apart from how your friends feel, neglecting them deprives you of an important resource. Good friends can be a valuable support during rough spots in your relationship. They may also be able to see things you don't—such as problems you're not willing to face or good things you've failed to appreciate.

Another problem with spending too much time together is that you or your partner may neglect your obligations. For example, your desire to be with your boyfriend or girlfriend may cause you to become careless about your school work, skip athletic practice, show up late for work, or miss a planned activity with your friends or family.

Finally, spending too much time with your boyfriend or girlfriend can take you away from people, activities, and interests that help you develop as a person. Couples can get to the point where they rely only on each other and don't interact with a wide variety of people. This can keep you from refining your interpersonal skills. It also robs you of the opportunity to find out more about yourself as you interact with others.

Giving up activities and interests has a similar effect. Couples who spend all their time together may miss out on knowledge and skills they might have picked up, as well as a chance to learn about themselves as they engage in those activities. They also close off avenues for self-expression.

Added Risk for Sex

Finally, if you're going steady or engaged, you're more likely to have sex. Steady or engaged couples usually spend more time alone, which provides both the opportunity and the temptation to have sex. What's more, steady or engaged couples are able to rationalize having sex on the grounds that "we love each other" or "we're going to get married anyway."

One such couple was Jack and

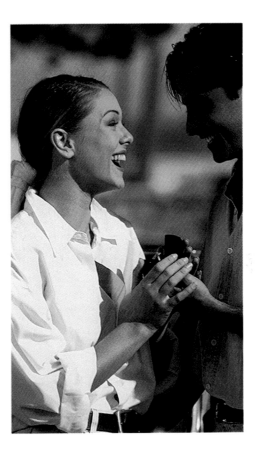

Leilani. Seniors in college, Jack and Leilani were planning to get married in the spring following their graduation. They were majoring in business and hoped to set up a consulting firm after they were married. Once they became engaged, the couple decided to have sex because, they said, they wanted to find out if they were "sexually compatible." They said they loved each other and rationalized that it was all right to have sex since they were engaged and knew they would be getting married.

A month before graduation, Leilani discovered that she had feelings for Art, another student in one of her classes. She broke her engagement with Jack,

CHOICES AND CONSEQUENCES

Premarital sex involves choices and consequences that affect every aspect of the human person.
What are some of the consequences of premarital sex now and in the future?

Choices	Saying No	Saying Yes	Consequences of Saying Yes

Physical Health	No change.	• Pregnancy:
		  - baby
		  - abortion
		  - adoption
		• STD/AIDS
		• Contraceptive side effects
			• STD affecting self and baby
			• Baby
			• Infertility

Mental/ Intellectual Life	• Maturity • Confidence • Self-esteem • Integrity • Educational goals pursued	• Self-centered • Closed-minded	• Sex is viewed as recreational and self-serving • Partners aren't respected and valued
Moral Character	• Formation of character • Consistent with one's beliefs • Value human beings	• Conflict of right and wrong • Treat others poorly, intentionally and unintentionally	• Indifferent toward values and those who have standards • Difficulty getting along with others • Raising children without values
Emotional Well-Being	• High self-worth • Able to channel sexual desires into nonsexual actions • Peace of mind	• Guilt • Depression • Rejection • Fear • Temporary feeling of love • Confusion	• Fooled into marrying wrong person • Distrust others • Difficulty maintaining relationships • Counseling • Self-hatred/jealousy
Social Growth	• Deeper understanding of others • Respected by self and others • Loss of a boyfriend or girlfriend	• Unwanted reputation • Temporary feeling of fitting in • No social standards • Attracting others with no standards	• Haunting reputation • Cohabitation instead of marriage • Cost to society, such as unwed teens with babies on welfare

Personal Goals and Dreams	• Unaffected short- and long-term goals
	• Ability to change plans at any time
		• Pregnancy:
		  -loss of education
		  -loss of adolescence
		  -child support payments
		  -money needed for raising a child or abortion
			• Formation of family and children jeopardized
			• Educational goals interrupted

started dating Art, and later moved in with him.

Jack and Leilani's wedding invitations were canceled, along with the couple's dreams and plans. Jack almost failed to graduate because of the emotional toll the breakup took on him. His biggest regret was that they didn't wait for marriage to have sex.

You can avoid sexual involvement during engagement by following the suggestions on dating given earlier in this chapter. Also, you can avoid the rationalizations by acknowledging that they *are* rationalizations—and that their purpose is to justify something you know is wrong. The very fact that you need to rationalize something is a strong indication that you know it's wrong. Once you realize that, you will look at rationalizations in an entirely different light. Instead of being persuaded by them, you can recognize them as warning signs urging you to say *no*.

Is It Really Love?

Quite often, relationships are based on infatuation rather than love. Infatuation may seem like love, and it's often intense, but there are several important differences. These differences can have an enormous impact on the quality of a romantic relationship and on whether you continue a relationship. Self-knowledge, being able to understand your own feelings and motivations, is essential to knowing whether to stay in and develop a relationship, or whether to let it come to an end.

The chart titled "Distinguishing Between Infatuation and Love" provides several clues for drawing this distinction. In the left column are questions you should ask about yourself, your partner, and your relationship. If most of your answers are like those in the far right column, your relationship is probably based on genuine love. On the other hand, if most of your answers are like those in the middle column, that's a sign your relationship is based on infatuation.

If the clues point to infatuation in your relationship, you need to be honest with yourself and with your partner. Sometimes giving your relationship

more time to develop will deepen the feelings. On the other hand, you may need to break off the relationship as a dating couple. That will free you both to get to know others, ideally someone with whom you can build a solid relationship based on love.

What If You've Already Gone Too Far?

Dating and romantic relationships can pose a particularly tough challenge if you've already had sex. You may feel that since you've already lost your virginity, there's no reason to abstain. If you've lost your self-respect, you may despair of ever getting it back again. And once you've had sex, it's harder to resist the temptation to do it again.

Although you'll never regain your physical virginity, you can regain both your self-control and your self-respect. Put another way, you may have lost your physical virginity, but you can still have secondary, or renewed, virginity by choosing to stop having sex and sticking to that decision until you're married.

Sticking to your decision may be tough, but you can do several things to make it easier to abstain from sex. Perhaps one of the most important things you can do is set clear standards for your future relationships—or your present one, if you're currently in one. Such standards could be similar to those mentioned earlier in this chapter:

- "I will keep myself pure for the person I marry."
- "I will not pet."
- "I will not be alone with my date in

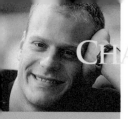

DISTINGUISHING BETWEEN INFATUATION AND LOVE		
Question to Ask	Clues to Look for: Infatuation	Clues to Look for: Love
1. What is my main interest? What attracts me most?	The person's physical appearance; things that register with my five senses.	The total personality; what's inside.
2. How many things attract me?	Few—though some may be strong.	Many or most.
3. How did the romance start?	Fast (hours or days).	Slowly (months or years).
4. How consistent is my level of interest?	Interest varies, comes and goes; many peaks and valleys; not consistent or predictable.	Evens out; gets to be dependable and consistent; can predict it.
5. What effect does the romance have on my personality?	Disorganized, destructive; I'm acting strangely; I'm not myself.	Organized, constructive; I'm a better person.
6. How does the relationship end?	Quickly, unless there's been mutually satisfying sex, which can prolong, but not save, the relationship.	Slowly, if at all; the relationship takes a long time to end; we'll never be quite the same.
7. How do I view my partner?	There's only one person in the world—my partner; my partner can do no wrong; I see my partner as faultless, idealizing him or her.	I'm realistic about my partner's strengths and weaknesses. I can admit my partner's faults, but I keep loving anyway.
8. How do others view our relationship? What's the attitude of friends and parents?	Few or none approves of the relationship.	Most or all approve. We get along well with each other's friends and parents.
9. What does distance (long separation) do to the relationship?	Withers away, dies; can't stand this added stress.	Survives; may even grow stronger.
10. How do quarrels affect the romance?	They get more frequent, more severe, and eventually kill the relationship.	They grow less frequent, less severe.
11. How do I feel about and refer to my relationship?	Much use of I/me/my; he/him/his; she/her/hers; little feeling of oneness.	Speak of we/us/our; feel and think as a unit, a pair; togetherness.
12. What's my ego response to the other?	Mainly selfish, conditional: "What does this do for me?"	Mainly unselfish, releasing; concerned equally for the other.
13. What's my overall attitude toward the other?	Attitude of taking; exploiting and using the other.	Attitude of giving, sharing; wanting to serve the other's needs and wants.
14. How much jealousy do I or my partner experience?	More frequent, more severe.	Less frequent, less severe.

my house or my date's."

- "I will not use alcohol or drugs."
- "I will not go to parties where people are drinking, taking drugs, or having sex."

If you're in a relationship, and you're being sexually intimate, stop. Depending on the relationship and the people involved, it may be best to end it. For some persons, backing up in a sexual relationship can be like trying to back their car up an icy hill. Other persons, through strength of character, prayer, and avoiding temptation, have been able to stop having sex and to develop a relationship based on intellectual, emotional, and spiritual intimacy.

Some other things you can do to help you abstain from sex are the following:

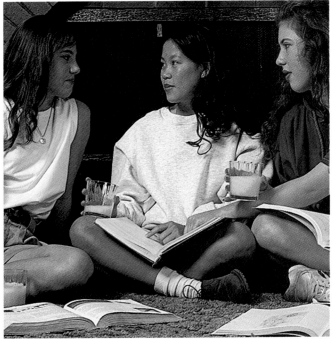

- Ask for support and encouragement from friends, family members, or others who share your values. Tell them about your commitment and ask them to hold you to it. They can help you live out your convictions.
- Make it clear by your actions that you are saying *no* to fooling around and petting. Follow the suggestions given earlier in this chapter for dressing appropriately. Avoid suggestive talk or teasing behavior. If your partner's hands start to roam, get up and go to a place where other people are present. Be assertive and consistent. Say *no* and stick to it.
- Avoid people, places, and situations that have led to sexual involvement in the past.
- Avoid sexually provocative magazines, movies, television programs, music, computer games, or Internet sites. Learn to distinguish between fantasy and reality. The media often portray sex outside marriage as simply a normal and pleasurable activity. But they fail to show the very real physical and emotional problems that go along with it. Remember that distinction when you watch movies or television, or listen to music.
- Put your energy into new hobbies and interests. This will keep you busy and help you stay away from compromising situations.
- Accept your past mistakes and learn from them. Forgive yourself and start over.
- Learn new ways of showing affection that don't arouse sexual feelings: write a poem, send inexpensive gifts, cook a favorite meal, pick some flowers.
- Cultivate new friendships. This is especially important if your old friends don't support your decision or are pressuring you to abandon it.
- Stand up for your choice. Many

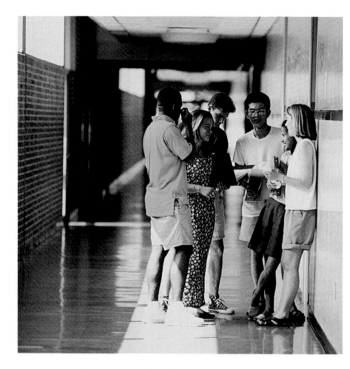

I met Ray at work. He was different from the others I had been dating. He seemed so kind and nice. He and I became friends right off. We started to date, then became boyfriend and girlfriend.

I, of course, wanted to have sex (because this was still part of a relationship—I had thought), but he was hesitant. He did end up having sex with me, but he seemed to change after we did.

He was so nice when we first started our relationship—he was the first guy to treat me so well. Now all he wanted to do was have sex. (I found out later that he was a virgin and that he gave up a lot of his morals to have sex with me.)

I wasn't liking this relationship. I was starting to see this sex before marriage for what it really was—a lie.

It was so hard to tell Ray that I didn't want to have sex anymore. After all, he gave up his virginity for me—so who was I to tell him we should stop having sex? He gave me an engagement ring to give me more of a feeling of commitment, but it didn't help.

He was getting more aggressive, and I was seeing that our relationship was nothing but sex. Two years into our relationship and with an engagement ring on my finger, I made the biggest step in my life. I broke up with him. I had to find out what real love was all about....

Three months later I saw Ray. We talked about what was happening, and I told him that I had changed. He realized

teens have joined others nationwide in pledging themselves to purity. Some young people wear a ring given to them by their parents; it symbolizes their commitment to save sex for marriage. Speaking out will help you be more serious about your decision and about changing. Other people may hear about it and make the same decision to remain pure until marriage.

Do you remember Susan, the young woman in chapter 2 who had sex with her boyfriend, Greg, and then with others to try to feel better after Greg broke up with her? She finally met someone she really cared about—Ray—but they too had sex. Eventually, however, she began to see things differently and chose secondary virginity, something anyone who has been sexually active can do. Here is the rest of her true story:

that he needed to change also.

We began seeing each other again. But from that point on we did not have sex. We began a beautiful relationship of communication and genuine friendship.

I never would have thought that letting go and seeking for true love would have given me so much joy. But now I am happily married to Ray, and the blessings that have come from our waiting until marriage to have sex have been worth it![2]

THE GOLDEN RULE

Claire is an eighteen-year-old senior and a virgin. She has been dating her boyfriend for six months. She is trying to decide whether to have sex with him on prom night. Claire is trusting that she won't get pregnant on the first and only time she plans to have sex before going off to college. She's also counting on her boyfriend's commitment if she does get pregnant. Claire approaches you with her problem.

- You are her best friend. What is your advice to her?
- You are her mother/father. What is your advice to her?
- You are her teacher. What is your advice to her?

Once you have answered these questions, ask yourself the following questions:
- What are the differences in your advice as friend, parent, and teacher?
- What is the same in your advice as friend, parent, and teacher?
- Should your advice as friend, parent, and teacher be basically the same?

Claire's health and well-being are at stake. True love is not expressed by sexual activity. Love is giving for the good of another person. Love does not expose the other person to unnecessary risk—like pregnancy, disease, or mental anguish. Birth control doesn't make sexual activity more loving; it simply changes the risk factor. Love refuses to hurt yourself or the other person.

If you are Claire's friend and are yourself sexually active, your advice will probably be different in each of the roles. Most likely you won't tell Claire not to have sex because you're doing the same thing. It will be difficult for you to encourage her to abstain from sex unless you are abstaining as well.

What if Claire was trying to decide about using cocaine? What would your advice be then? Your response should be to discourage Claire from using cocaine. Cocaine use is never good. Like people who engage in premarital sex,

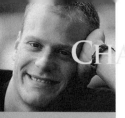

people who use cocaine expose themselves and others to unnecessary risks.

An enabler is someone who is aware of a friend's problem but allows, condones, or enables the behavior that's causing the problem to continue anyway. Enablers typically either ignore a problem, rationalize it, or deny that it exists.

Enablers are not true friends. True friends face problems squarely by showing tough love. Tough love is the willingness to stand up to friends when they are hurting themselves or others, even at the risk of losing the friendship.

TESTING A SEXUAL RELATIONSHIP

What if an unmarried couple is sexually active and one of the partners asks the other to stop having sex? How would being infatuated or being in love affect the other partner's reaction? Here are some possible reactions:

- The other partner does not want to stop having sex.
- The other partner says that not having sex will hurt the relationship.
- The other partner decides to end the relationship (thus indicating that he or she did not really love the partner).
- The other partner agrees at first but after some time begins to complain about missing sexual intimacy.
- The other partner is relieved and feels better about the relationship.

If the other partner insists on continuing to have sex, then this person is not really concerned about the partner's well-being. Sex can be addictive. If you're addicted to sex, you need to break this habit and learn a new one: sexual self-control. It's definitely possible to do so, and there are great rewards.

On the other hand, if a partner is not willing to unlearn an unhealthy habit, he or she will continue to exploit the other person. Such a relationship needs to end immediately. Exploitative sex never provides the foundation for a healthy relationship. Exploitative sex, by rejecting self-control, cheapens a relationship and belittles the partner.

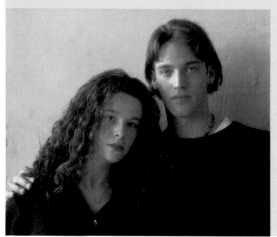

Love wants what is best for the other person. Love never puts anyone at unnecessary risk of pregnancy, disease, or heartache. Love is giving for the good of another. Love—true love—always looks out for other people's emotional, physical, and moral well-being.

If you're involved in a sexual

relationship and want to stop, you need to develop cessation skills. Cessation skills set guidelines that help a person regain self-control by abstaining from a particular behavior, such as premarital sex, drug use, viewing pornography, or violence. The following cessation skills can help young people regain sexual self-control:

1. **Give reasons for your decision.** Examples include:
   - I want to feel more self-respect instead of feeling used.
   - It's straining my relationship with friends and family members.
   - The health risks are too high.
   - I never really know the sexual history of another person.

2. **Reinforce the decision by your behavior.**
   - Avoid places and people that cause you to slip.
   - Body language can give a strong NO message.
   - Don't flirt with the unhealthy behavior, thinking you're strong enough to abstain from it.

3. **Plan alternatives.**
   - Associate with friends who will support your healthy behaviors.
   - Begin working out and exercising.
   - Discuss other ways of finding pleasure that are both healthy and positive.

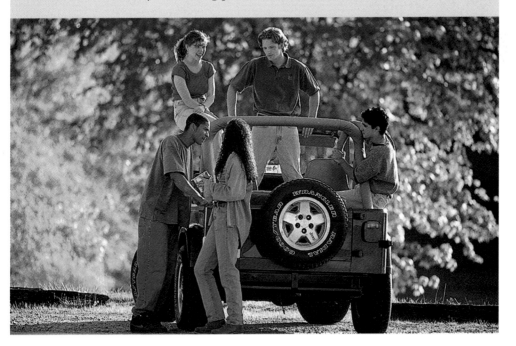

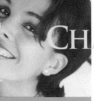

4. Stick to your decision to change.
- Be assertive when you are pressured.
- Exercise self-control when you are pressured.
- Point out the problems of engaging in unhealthy behaviors.
- Keep in mind the responsibilities you have both as a student and as a son or daughter living at home.
- Respect yourself and demand respect from others.

By practicing these cessation skills and regaining sexual self-control, you put yourself back on the path to becoming a mature adult. Twelve-year-olds are capable of having sex, but that doesn't make them mature men and women. Mature adults respect themselves and others by exercising self-control and responsibility.

EXAMINING YOUR CHARACTER AND LEVEL OF SEXUAL MATURITY

Controlling one's desires presents a tough challenge in today's culture, which encourages immediate gratification rather than self-control. Movies, videos, music, and advertising frequently glamorize premarital sex and extramarital affairs. Besides the media, young people are surrounded by negative adult role models who casually engage in uncommitted sexual relationships.

Sexual behavior outside a committed and loving lifetime relationship undermines character and exploits others for personal pleasure. Premature sexual activity is destructive, both physically and emotionally. Many young people today take serious, unnecessary risks with their own and another person's health by engaging in premarital sex.

In the following pages you will have an opportunity to examine your character and level of sexual maturity. Read each statement in the following tables.

On a separate sheet of paper write down the number from the column that best describes how often your behavior is consistent with the statement. After you do that for every statement in a given table, add up the numbers you've written down. The total is your overall rating for the character trait printed at the top of the table.

After you've taken this survey, encourage someone you know and trust—perhaps a coach or friend—to take the survey and evaluate your character. See how your answers compare. Discuss the results.

A score of 25–30 for a given table indicates that you usually exemplify that particular character trait in your dating relationships. Congratulations! Keep up the good work. A score of 20–24 indicates that you are doing well but there is some room for growth. Developing positive habits requires perseverance. A score of 10–19 suggests that you need to improve your character. It will take self-control and determination to do so, but good character in your dating relationships is never out of reach.

HONESTY	ALWAYS	SOMETIMES	NEVER
1. Are you honest with yourself about how you feel about the person you're dating?	3	2	1
2. Would you tell your partner if you had a sexually transmitted disease?	3	2	1
3. Are you honest with your date if you don't want to have sex?	3	2	1
4. Would you tell someone you love him/her just to have sex?	1	2	3
5. Would you tell your parents if you were sexually active?	3	2	1
6. Would you be honest enough with yourself to ask an adult, a counselor, or a parent for help in saying no to sex?	3	2	1
7. Can you tell your partner that you no longer want to have sex?	3	2	1
8. If you think you have an STD, are you willing to get a checkup?	3	2	1
9. Do you lie to your friends about having sex?	1	2	3
10. Would you remain in a relationship just to have sex?	1	2	3

Your overall Honesty rating: _____

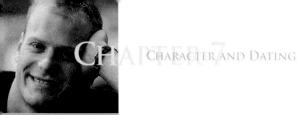

RESPECT	ALWAYS	SOMETIMES	NEVER
1. If sexually active, would you respect your partner's wishes to stop having sex?	3	2	1
2. Would you respect your parent's instruction not to have sex?	3	2	1
3. Would you ridicule your friends if they wanted to practice abstinence?	1	2	3
4. Would you dress provocatively to get dates?	1	2	3
5. Would you respect your partner's wishes not to have sex?	3	2	1
6. Would you jeopardize someone else's future reproductive health for your personal gratification?	1	2	3
7. Would you try to get someone drunk in order to have sex?	1	2	3
8. Is it all right to pressure someone into having sex?	1	2	3
9. Would you date someone seriously if that person would not have had sex prior to marriage?	3	2	1
10. Is premarital sex all right as long as there's no pregnancy because of it?	1	2	3

Your overall Respect rating: _____

COURAGE	ALWAYS	SOMETIMES	NEVER
1. Could you tell your partner that you want to stop making out, petting, or having sex?	3	2	1
2. Would you seek medical attention if you thought you had an STD?	3	2	1
3. Would you seek advice from your parents if you had been hurt in a relationship?	3	2	1
4. Can you tell your sexually active friends that premarital sex is not a good idea?	3	2	1
5. Would you stop having sex until marriage even if your partner didn't want to?	3	2	1
6. Would you be willing to wait to have sex until marriage even though others may laugh at you?	3	2	1
7. Can you confront sexually active friends when they are hurting others?	3	2	1
8. Are you able to ask for help when you want to stop having sex?	3	2	1
9. Would you choose not to view a sexually explicit movie even if your friends were doing it?	3	2	1
10. Can you say no to premarital sex and mean it?	3	2	1

Your overall Courage rating: _____

SELF-DISCIPLINE	ALWAYS	SOMETIMES	NEVER
1. Do your sexual feelings control your actions?	1	2	3
2. Can you turn down sex?	3	2	1
3. If sexually aroused, do you pressure your date into having sex?	1	2	3
4. Do you avoid drinking on a date?	3	2	1
5. Are you willing to wait to have sex until marriage?	3	2	1
6. Can you regain your sexual self-control?	3	2	1
7. Do you read pornographic material?	1	2	3
8. Do you avoid touching your date in a sexual manner?	3	2	1
9. Do you think sexual feelings are controllable?	3	2	1
10. Are you willing not to view sexually explicit forms of media, including TV shows, videos, or movies?	3	2	1

Your overall Self-Discipline rating: _____

RESPONSIBILITY	ALWAYS	SOMETIMES	NEVER
1. Are you ready for your date on time?	3	2	1
2. Do you drink or do drugs while on a date?	1	2	3
3. Do you think any sexual activity short of full sexual intercourse is all right?	1	2	3
4. If pregnancy occurs, would you approve an abortion?	1	2	3
5. Do you consider sexual self-control a good thing?	3	2	1
6. Would you explain to your younger siblings the advantages of abstinence?	3	2	1
7. Do you plan a date in advance so you can avoid opportunities for sexual activity?	3	2	1
8. Do you treat dating as a step toward marriage?	3	2	1
9. Do you keep the agreements and promises you make to the person you're dating?	3	2	1
10. Can you accept correction if you've behaved badly on a date?	3	2	1

Your overall Responsibility rating: _____

KINDNESS	ALWAYS	SOMETIMES	NEVER
1. Would you avoid premarital sex to protect the future well-being of your date?	3	2	1
2. Are you concerned about your date's physical and emotional health?	3	2	1
3. Do you ignore your date's request not to be sexually active?	1	2	3
4. Do you encourage your friends who want to stay virgins until they marry?	3	2	1
5. Do you make fun of those who are not sexually active?	1	2	3
6. Are you willing to speak to a friend about the benefits of abstinence?	3	2	1
7. Are you an example of abstinence for your little brother or sister?	3	2	1
8. In the next year, do you expect to be sexually involved with someone?	1	2	3
9. After spending time or money with someone, do you get angry if it doesn't lead to sex?	1	2	3
10. Do you actively look for ways to make your date happy instead of just looking out for yourself?	3	2	1

Your overall Kindness rating: _____

1. Many young people who have committed themselves to sexual purity have learned the hard way that sex without a lifelong commitment is empty. Does dating imply a serious enough commitment to engage in a sexual relationship?

2. Consider the following statement: "I look forward to the day I can look my spouse in the face and say, 'I loved you before I even knew you. I saved myself just for you.'" Would you like to hear these words from your future spouse? Would you like your future spouse to hear them from you?

3. Many young people engage in sex because of low self-esteem. To feel good about themselves, they cling to a sexual partner even when there's no real commitment. How can controlling one's sexual desires and regaining sexual self-control increase one's self-worth?

4. Steady dating and teen pregnancy often go hand in hand. Why do you think this happens?

5. Couples who cohabit—that is, live together outside of marriage—sometimes end up getting married. But when they do, they tend to experience greater marital conflict and poorer communication than married couples who never cohabited.[3] Why do you think this happens? Discuss the following quote from Nancy Moore Clatworthy, a professor of sociology at Ohio State University, who studied married couples who lived together before marriage:

   Among the couples who had married and lived together first, the most common problems were in the areas of adjustment, happiness, and respect. For instance, the couples were asked to check off the degree of respect. Those who had married first and not lived together had a higher degree of respect than those who had lived together.

   The couples were asked how often did they fantasize about breaking off with their spouse. One of the answers to this question was "often." The only people who checked that answer had lived together before they were married.[4]

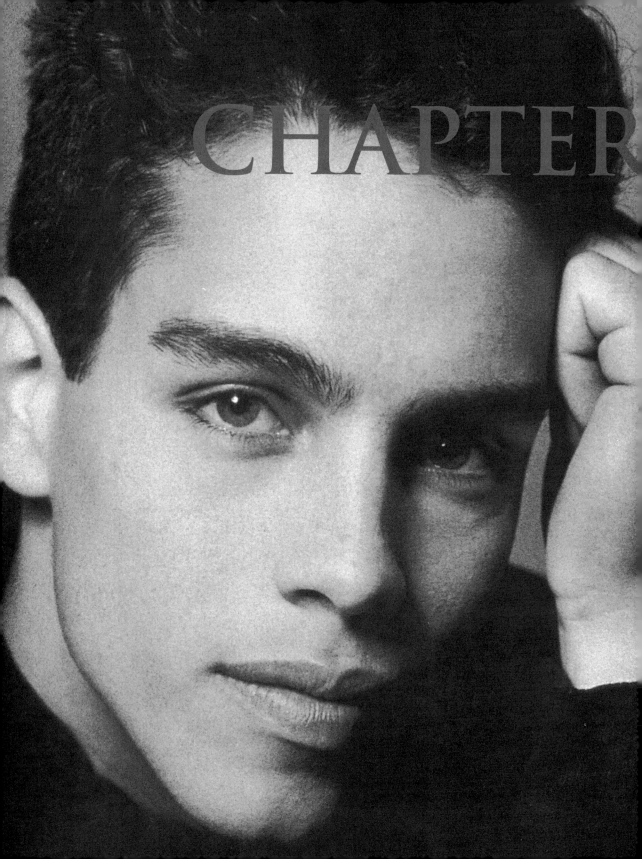

CHAPTER

8

Marriage turns out to be the best way to have

regular sex and the best way to have a happy

sex life.

CHARACTER AND MARRIAGE

-Sex in America, A Definitive Survey, 1994[†]

George was like most of the other boys in high school. He liked girls—and one in particular. He thought she liked him, but she was dating other boys besides him.

After George got to college, he was startled to hear that she had married someone else. He found out later that they had to get married—she was pregnant. George was crushed. He didn't think he would love another girl again.

In college he dated, but not seriously. "Then I met an unusual girl at a party," he says. "She was skinny and had bushy eyebrows. I wasn't particularly attracted to her, but I noticed that she was different—quiet and ladylike."

George enjoyed being with Laura, and they started dating.

"She had high principles. She wouldn't let me kiss her," he says.

In time Laura decided that George was the one she'd been looking for.

"That first kiss was historic!" says George. "It really meant something to both of us."

Before long they both knew they loved each other. They talked about marrying when George finished college. He graduated from Georgia Tech with an engineering degree, received a commission in the navy, and married Laura—all in three days.

"Neither my wife nor I had any previous sexual experience before we got married. We were both virgins, so we felt pretty awkward. But we were so in love that it didn't matter. One wonderful thing about our marriage," he adds, "was that neither of us brought any 'baggage' into the marriage from previous sexual experiences."

George and Laura were married in May 1942 when America was at war. They were together for only four weeks before he had to ship out to the Pacific Ocean to serve on board a cruiser.

"My ship was torpedoed in a night battle at Guadalcanal, and we went to Australia for repairs. There were plenty of 'available' women in Australia. Many of the married guys on our ship spent their liberty time ashore shacking up with a woman, but I didn't go with them. Back home my precious young wife, who loved me with all her heart, was waiting for me. That meant something to me."

George returned to the States twice

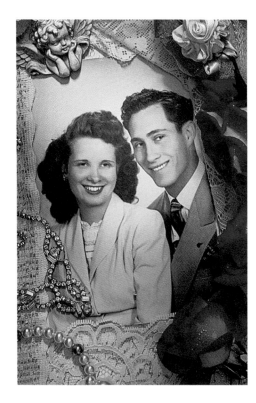

Devastated by this tragedy, George says that their love brought them through.

George and Laura have five children and ten grandchildren. "We love them all, and our love for each other is stronger than ever," he says.[1]

Both George and Laura knew that marriage was special—so special that they held off sex until they were married. Not only that, but George showed how much he valued his marriage and his new wife by staying faithful to her even when they were apart. While other men gave in to loneliness and temptation, George did not.

In this chapter we'll look at marriage, what it is and how it benefits husbands, wives, and children. We'll also look at ways your character can affect you, whether you choose to remain single or to marry. And we'll examine some of the advantages of saving sex until marriage.

during the war years to see his wife. It wasn't easy for the young couple to be separated.

"What a thrill it was to come home after the war to be with my wife. This time she had our baby boy in her arms. How wonderful it was to be with my wife and son!"

Throughout the years George and Laura's love for one another grew stronger. They experienced some difficult times. Their son Bruce was killed in an accident when he was seven.

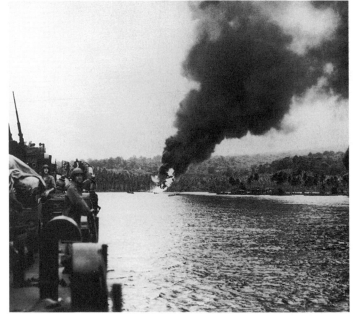

What Is Marriage?

Most people in our culture think of marriage as an intimate and private relationship between a man and a woman—a relationship in which society approves sexual intercourse and encourages childbearing.

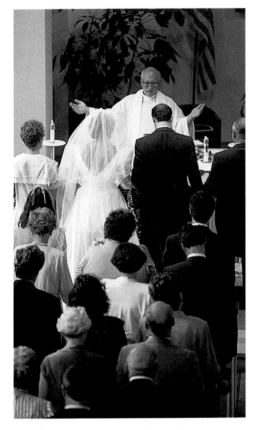

Although marriage has this private aspect, it also has some very public aspects. For example, consider the following facts about marriage in our society:

- Marriages in our society are almost always brought into being in a formal ceremony attended by witnesses.[2]
- This ceremony may be conducted only by certain officials, such as judges, clerks of the court, licensed ministers, priests, or rabbis.
- Each marriage must be properly registered in the county where the ceremony occurred.
- Married couples must go through a formal divorce to end their marriage.

Why all the requirements? Marriage turns unrelated people into family members—with all the rights and obligations that family members have.

One very important obligation family members have is to take care of each other and look out for each other's welfare. When one partner becomes sick or injured, for instance, the first person to pick up the slack and tend to that partner's needs is the other partner.

Marriage partners are also expected to share their resources and provide for each other in a way that unmarried couples are not. In fact, "nonsupport" (also called "refusal to provide" or "gross neglect of duty") is considered grounds for divorce in some states.[3] This occurs when one spouse—usually the husband—is able to provide for the other but persistently refuses to do so.

In addition to these obligations, marriage also gives each partner several important legal rights, including the right to:

- make medical decisions about one's spouse if that spouse becomes seriously ill or injured;
- collect pension, disability, unemployment, Social Security, and veteran's benefits;
- receive the other spouse's estate if that spouse dies without leaving a will; and
- sue a third party for the wrongful death of the other spouse.

Even so, the consequences of marriage go beyond the relationship between husband and wife. Besides uniting husband and wife, marriage also unites the husband to the couple's children. Compare this with two unmarried people having sex—if the woman gets pregnant, the man may refuse to acknowledge the child as his own.

Sexual intercourse is a private, intimate event. A wedding ceremony, on the other hand, is a very public event. By taking part in that ceremony, the husband publicly acknowledges having a sexual relationship with his wife and thus accepts responsibility for any children the couple may conceive. Once married, he cannot easily refuse to acknowledge his children.

But the consequences of marriage don't stop with the immediate family. Marriage not only unites the husband, wife, and children, but also places them in a larger network of family relationships. The husband becomes part of the wife's family, and the wife becomes part of the husband's. Their children, too, become part of that network.

This has important implications for the husband, wife, and children because it opens more resources for them to draw on. As anthropologist David Murray points out:

> We do not hope to receive tuition, childcare, or a kidney from a business associate, but we do from relatives. Marriage is that device which extends to us a social security network of obligated kin. As such, marriages are political and economic affairs, and are regarded by most people of the world as far too important to be left in the hands of personal attraction. For many traditional cultures, marriage may contain romance, but the institution serves primarily to "arrange" the structure of society.[4]

Finally, in addition to its personal, social, and legal dimensions, marriage has a religious dimension for many people. Many religions, including

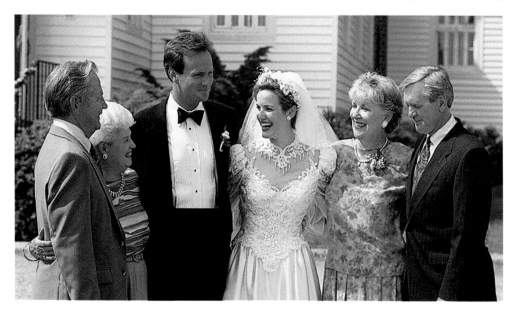

Christianity, Islam, and Judaism, teach that marriage was originally established by God and that married people are ultimately accountable to God for their conduct in the marriage relationship. That accountability is underscored in the sacred writings of many religions, as well as in religious wedding ceremonies, during which both the husband and wife make sacred vows.

WEDDING TRADITIONS

The word *wedding* comes from the old English word *wed*, which means "promise" or "pledge." Common wedding traditions that are used today include the following:

- **Bride's White Dress and Veil:** The bride wears a white dress and veil to symbolize her innocence and purity.
- **Exchange of Rings:** A circle has no beginning and no end, and symbolizes eternity. The fourth finger of the left hand is chosen as the ring finger because, according to legend, a vein or nerve runs from that finger to the heart.

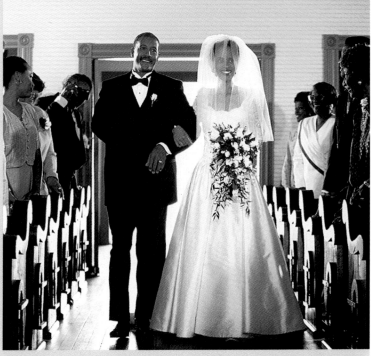

- **Throwing Rice:** Throwing rice at a newly married couple symbolizes fertility and expresses the hope that the couple will be blessed with children.

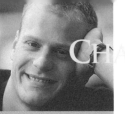

BENEFITS OF MARRIAGE

In addition to its personal, social, legal, and religious dimensions, marriage also provides great practical benefits to husbands and wives, to fathers in particular, and to the children.

BENEFITS OF MARRIAGE TO HUSBANDS AND WIVES

Married people have better sex. According to the most comprehensive survey of sexual practices in America, "having one sex partner is more rewarding in terms of physical pleasure and emotional satisfaction than having more than one partner, and it is particularly rewarding if that single partner is a marriage partner.... A monogamous sexual partnership embedded in a formal marriage evidently produces the greatest satisfaction and pleasure."[5]

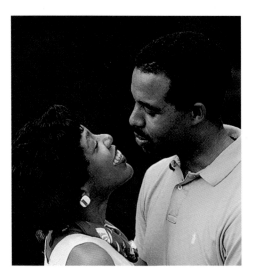

One explanation the researchers offer is that "the longer the partnership is likely to last, and the more commitment one has to that partnership, the greater is the incentive to learn what pleases that partner, what excites, what frustrates, what angers—in short, what works sexually and what does not. We should thus expect to see that partnerships characterized by commitment and long-term prospects would be relatively successful in achieving sexual satisfaction."[6]

But there's more to it than that. Married sex is intrinsically more meaningful than uncommitted sex. Consider what our bodies are saying in the act of sexual intercourse. Sexual intercourse says, "I give myself to you completely." In marriage, that's really true; without marriage, it's not. Sexual union in marriage expresses the complete commitment a man and a woman have made to each other. They join their bodies because they've joined their lives. That is why sex has more meaning and is more fulfilling within marriage.

Marriage offers another big advantage: freedom from the painful emotional baggage that accompanies unmarried sex (see chapter 6). This includes:

- fear of unwed pregnancy;
- fear of sexually transmitted disease;
- guilt and depression about the act itself, with the accompanying fear of being caught;
- guilt about deceiving parents or others;
- fear of being "used" by others;
- regret and self-reproach; and
- loss of self-respect.

Freedom from this baggage makes it easier for both partners to focus on the pleasure of sex, instead of being distracted by other issues.

Married men are also more fulfilled sexually than single men. One study reports that married men have sex twice as often each month as single men. Married men described the quality of that sex as more emotionally and physically satisfying than unmarried men did.[7]

Finally, marriage improves sex by enhancing both partners' sense of security. This is especially true for women. Psychiatrist David Larson points out that women are more likely to enjoy sex "when they feel secure, loved, and trusting that their man is around to stay. Without a doubt, marriage provides a foundation that increases the odds a woman will be able to risk a level of vulnerability that goes beyond the ability to participate in the act but enables her to 'let go.'"[8]

Mark and Lisa, both in their mid-twenties, had been married for two and a half years and were expecting their first child. They had waited until they were married to have sex.

"Sex is an essential part of marriage," Mark says, "but it isn't the reason for marriage. You don't get married in order to have sex. You get married in order to be united to another person."[9]

Married people are generally healthier than unmarried adults. Married men, in particular, experience better physical health than men who are single, divorced, or widowed. The longer the marriage, the greater the benefits.[10] Men who are not married exhibit more harmful behaviors, such as fighting, accidents, and excessive drinking. Because of increased alcoholism, single men have a three times greater chance of dying from cirrhosis of the liver than married men. In terms of reduced life expectancy, it's more dangerous for a man to be unmarried than to weigh too much, smoke, or have heart disease or cancer.[11]

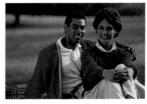

Members of intact families have higher overall health ratings than family members who are divorced.[12] This is also true for divorced women, who report having poorer health than married women. Age is not a factor here since married people are on average slightly older than those who are divorced.[13]

As a group, both men and women who are divorced or separated experience higher rates of sickness, disability, mental difficulties, and death than do men and women who are married. This is true for whites and nonwhites in all age categories over twenty.[14]

Married people experience better mental health than unmarried people. Married people also reap mental health benefits. Married people are less likely to develop schizophrenia or be admitted to mental hospitals than unmarried people.[15]

According to family sociologist David Popenoe, married people find that happiness comes not from money, but from the warm, intimate, and lasting relationship they develop with their spouse. In fact, studies have found that "nearly 40 percent of married adults report being 'very happy,'" while less than 25 percent of single adults report the same. Being fulfilled in marriage and having a satisfying family life is the "strongest single overall predictor of personal well-being."[16]

Although both men and women benefit from a good marriage, men benefit especially. As social psychologist Angus Campbell notes, "Men appear to suffer more from the absence of a wife than women do from the absence of a husband."[17] This is because women are usually more caring and nurturing than men, and thus are better at managing social relationships. Men consider their best friend to be their spouse more often than women do.[18]

Married people live longer than people who are divorced or separated. People who live with their mates live significantly longer than people who live by themselves or with someone who is not a marriage partner. Whether or not a marriage partner is present is the key factor.[19] Other research has shown that married men live longer than men who are single, divorced, or widowed.[20]

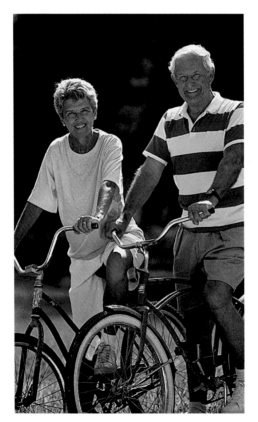

Married people are less prone to suicide. Empirical data going back to the nineteenth century show that suicide rates are lower among married people than among those who are divorced, widowed, or never married.[21] A solid family unites and strengthens the individual members, giving them a greater sense of purpose and less of a desire to end their lives.

Unmarried people, of course, can—and do—lead healthy, productive, and fulfilling lives. Indeed, some people feel "called" to the vocation of a single life as the best way to live out their deepest values and beliefs. Leading a life of character means being true to your inner convictions and caring for others, regardless of whether you decide to stay single or get married.

Married people experience greater satisfaction in life than single people.[22] For example, married men experience greater success on their jobs. One study showed that supervisors gave married men better performance evaluations than single men, thereby increasing their chances for promotion and better wages.[23]

Sociologist Catherine E. Ross sums up the benefits of marriage this way: "The positive effect of marriage on well-being is strong and consistent."[24]

DOES LIVING TOGETHER HELP?

But just living together without marriage doesn't improve a person's life. The relationships of couples who simply live together are not as healthy as those of married couples, reports one study. Their relationships are less stable and marked by more disagreement.[25]

Violence is significantly greater among couples who live together without

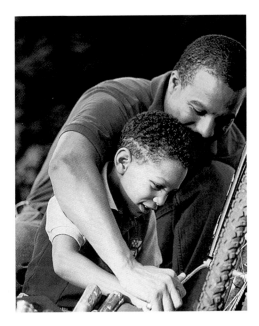

wedding vows. In one study, cohabiting couples were twice as likely to be violent as married couples, and the violence was five times more severe among cohabitants than among married people.[26]

People who merely live together are more likely to get depressed than those who are married.[27]

Couples who live together before marriage are more likely to have problems with drugs, alcohol, and sexual infidelity than those couples who do not live together first.

Cohabiting couples and couples who live together before they marry break up 50 to 100 percent more often than couples who get married without first living together.[28] Also, women who live with their future spouses before marriage are almost 80 percent more likely to end up in a broken relationship than women who do not cohabit.[29]

Marriage offers benefits to husbands and wives that are unmatched by any other form of relationship.

BENEFITS OF MARRIAGE TO FATHERS

Being a father also has its rewards. As family sociologist David Popenoe observes, fatherhood is "one of the most deeply satisfying and meaningful of life's endeavors."[30] It helps men see what's really important and enables them to feel part of other close relationships across generations. They learn such important virtues as compassion, kindness, patience, generosity, and unselfishness.[31]

As fatherhood expert Ross D. Parke puts it, "Fathering [is] good for men as well as for children."[32] Research shows that fathers who take an active role in raising their children fare better on their jobs, in their marriages, and in preparing the next generation.[33]

Research also shows that among men who marry, the happiest, most fulfilled men are fathers who have grown children and are still living with their wives. They tend to view their overall health as generally quite good. By contrast, those who are the unhappiest and least fulfilled are the men who do not live with their children and are not active in family life.[34]

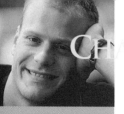

THE IMPORTANCE OF FATHERS

In *Life Without Father*, sociologist David Popenoe summarizes years of research about the importance of fathers:

- There is no substitute for fathers raising children. Most children profit greatly from living with a father who takes an active part in their lives. On the other hand, children who do not live with their fathers face significant disadvantages.

- Children need a mother and a father who are committed to working together for their good and give them consistent love and attention they can count on—at least while they are growing up.

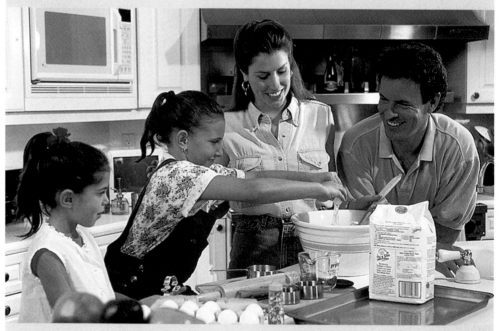

- Men need marriage to be good parents. A man is more likely to stay with the mother of his children if he is married to her. Fathers and mothers need encouragement from cultural, social, and economic sources to help them remain in their marriages.

- It's important for fathers to consider their children's feelings. Children need to feel special. They need to feel love and acceptance from their fathers.

- There is no substitute for biological fathers. Biological fathers are more likely to care deeply about their own children than nonbiological fathers, such as temporary boyfriends or stepfathers.[35]

Two parents can provide more resources than one.

The most obvious advantage of two-parent households is that they can provide more resources than a single parent. Having both a mother and a father at home usually means that there are two people present who can earn a living and care for the children instead of just one.

That makes an enormous difference in the children's standard of living. Children who live with only their mothers, which occurs in the vast majority of single-parent households, are far more likely to be poor than children in two-parent households. The United States Census Bureau reports that although only 18 percent of all families in the nation are headed by a woman householder with no spouse present, 54 percent of all *poor* families are headed by such a householder.[36]

The impact on young children is especially hard. Although only 11 percent of all children under age six living in married-couple families are poor, almost 62 percent of those living only with their mothers are poor.[37]

The additional resources that a two-parent family offers, however, are not merely economic. As David Popenoe points out:

> Childrearing is a demanding, stressful, and often exhausting activity that continues nonstop for at least eighteen years. Two adults can not only support and [relieve] one another; they can help counteract each other's deficiencies and contribute to each other's strengths. Two adults will invariably bring different skills and perspectives to a child....."[38]

Two parents provide a larger network of relatives.

Marriage places parents and children within a larger network of family relationships. Children are not only the parents' sons and daughters, but also someone else's cousins, nieces, nephews, and grandchildren. This provides children with resources from their parents as well as from other relatives. As anthropologist David Murray observes:

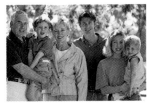

> Married couples, more than single parents, have parents and grandparents as a resource. House loans, emergency aid, car payments, cash gifts, and job opportunities come disproportionately from these relatives. Over one-fourth of all new home purchases depend upon gifts from parents. The gifts provided at a formal wedding assist a couple, as will the bestowal of an inheritance upon the eventual death of the parents. There is little question but that having four parents and eight grandparents attached to every marriage broadens the base of economic support....[39]

These same benefits, of course, extend to the couple's children.

A larger extended family means there are more people who care about the children. David Murray points out that these relationships are important for promoting moral action, a fact recognized in many cultures:

> The worst characterization the Navajo can offer of a thoughtless, deviant man is the charge that "he acts as if he has no relatives"....
>
> A man with no relatives, the Navajo feel, is a man with no concern for the shame or honor that his behavior might

bring upon those he loves. He acts, there-fore, without control or humanity....

We see a similar phenomenon in mod-ern America. People concerned about the reactions of relatives behave differently from people who are...anonymous strangers. The husband at a distant con-vention or the tourist abroad may do things under the cover of anonymity that would bring embarrassment were they done in front of one's mother, wife, chil-dren, or in-laws.[40]

Higher educational attainment. Chil-dren and adolescents who grow up with their fathers in the home, especially in the early years, experience fewer educa-tional problems. Research shows that they are more likely to:

- be proficient in school. Children from intact families score higher on intelligence tests and earn higher grades.[41]

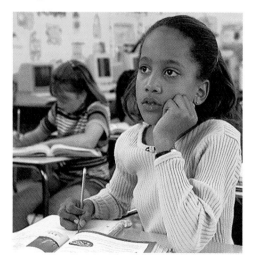

- achieve a higher level of education. Children from intact families stay in school longer, earning more diplomas and degrees.[42]

- experience fewer discipline prob-lems in school. One study showed that 35 percent of students who reside with both parents experi-enced school discipline problems, whereas 47 percent of students who reside with only their mothers experienced such problems.[43]

- avoid being suspended or expelled from school. That same study found that 27 percent of students from single-parent families were in dan-ger of being suspended from school compared to 19.6 percent of stu-dents from intact families.[44] In another study, 70 percent of seven-teen thousand children who did not live with their biological fathers were at greater risk of being expelled than children who were raised in a two-parent home.[45]

- be promoted each year to the next grade. In that same study of seven-teen thousand children, 40 percent of the children who did not live with their biological fathers were at greater risk of staying behind a year in school than children from two-parent families.[46]

- finish school. Children from intact families are twice as likely to graduate from school as children of divorce.[47]

Less risk of substance abuse. Children without a father in the home are not only more likely to use tobacco, alcohol, and drugs, but also to start using these substances earlier than children from intact families.[48]

Children from intact marriages are healthier physically and emotionally. In a report titled *Fatherhood and Family Health,* the Virginia Department of

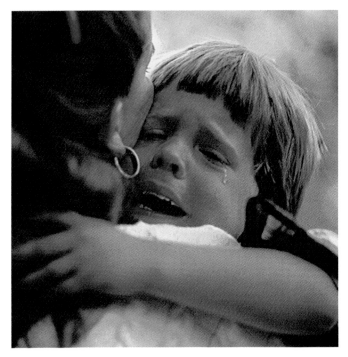

ward off disease.[49]

On the other hand, children who do not live with their biological fathers:

- have generally poorer physical health.[50] Children in single-parent families had a 20 to 35 percent greater risk of disease than children in two-parent families.[51]
- have more frequent headaches.[52]
- have more speech defects.[53]
- experience more emotional and behavioral problems.[54]
- receive more treatment from psychiatric and mental health professionals.[55]

Health notes that children who live with their biological fathers have better health than children who do not live with their biological fathers. They appear to have stronger immune systems and are therefore better able to

- risk being injured in accidents 20 to 30 percent more often than children who lived with their biological parents.[56]
- have a 50 percent greater risk of suffering from asthma.

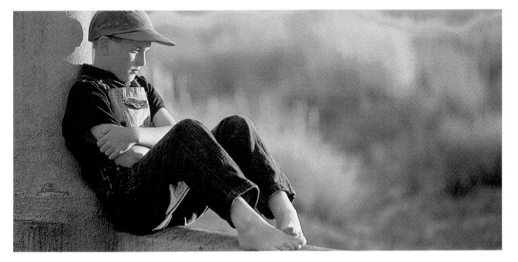

Divorce produces very severe and long-lasting effects on the people involved, but especially on children, says Judith Wallerstein, director of the Center for the Family in Transition. In her research she found that even six years following a divorce, a significant number of children were still experiencing behavioral and emotional problems connected with the divorce. These problems included irritability, impulsiveness, anxiety, and insecurity.[57]

According to Dr. Wallerstein, a significant number of the children who were age four when their parents divorced experienced serious disadvantages by the time they reached adolescence. Many had not learned to control their aggressive feelings or their tendency to withdraw from social situations.[58]

Ten years after the divorce almost 50 percent of the children were still anxious, achieving below their potential, critical of themselves, and frequently angry. They felt the divorce forced them to grow up too fast. They were anxious about what would happen to them, whether they might be abandoned, whether their parents could deal with their problems. Conflicts unresolved by the divorce only make matters worse. As one child remarked, "I wish I was dead. Then they wouldn't have to fight anymore."[59]

Less risk of teen pregnancy. When both parents are involved in the lives of their children, teen preg-

nancy occurs less frequently.

According to one study, a girl who has grown up in a single-parent home is over two and a half times more likely to conceive a child out of wedlock and over two times more likely to give birth as a teen than a girl from an intact family. If she marries, she has almost twice as great a chance of getting divorced as a girl who has grown up in a two-parent home.[60]

These statistics continue to hold for low-income families on welfare. Girls from low-income families who grow up without their fathers are more than twice as likely to give birth without being married as girls from low-income families who grow up with their fathers.[61] The father's presence makes a significant difference for families on welfare.

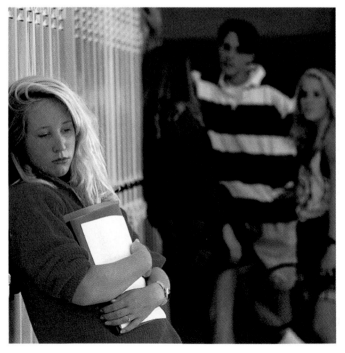

Lower risk of delinquency and crime. Although mothers may set community standards, fathers enforce them. Fatherless communities lack the men who will confront young people that go astray, or who will protect their communities from outside threats, such as gangs. They also lack the men who will hold other men responsible for fulfilling their roles as fathers. The presence of fathers helps bring peace to a neighborhood.[62]

Young people between the ages of twelve and twenty who live in single-parent homes often commit violent crimes and robberies.[63]

Delinquency occurs 10 to 15 percent more often among children from broken homes than among children from intact homes. Neither sex nor race makes a difference here. Growing up in a broken home has the same negative effect on a child, whether male or female, black or white.[64]

Seventy percent of the juveniles who reach state reform institutions were raised by one parent or no parents.[65]

Adolescents face many temptations to engage in at-risk health behaviors—for example, using drugs or engaging in premarital sex. Family environment is one of the key factors in avoiding these behaviors. Studies indicate that the presence of a father for boys and a mother for girls can reduce at-risk behaviors by giving the adolescents a strong role model to follow.[66]

Although most people like to think that nothing bad can happen to them, adolescents are especially guilty of this way of thinking. "It'll never happen to me" is a common response to warnings against pregnancy or being infected with sexually transmitted diseases (which is not to say, however, that having a child is the same as having a disease). Having a caring father and a caring mother in the home helps a child grow up with a clearer grasp of reality.

Lower risk of running away. Teenagers who run away from home most frequently come from homes with a stepparent, and most infrequently from homes with intact families where the biological father and mother are present.[67]

Lower risk of suicide. Children who grow up with fathers have a lower risk of committing suicide than children who grow up without fathers.[68]

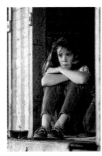

CHARACTER MATTERS

In chapter 7 we looked at the role character plays in dating. As important as it is for dating, character plays an even more important role in marriage. When you marry someone, you are no longer responsible for just your own welfare, but for the welfare of your spouse and, eventually, of your children.

What's more, your lives are joined in very practical ways. You share not only a bed, but also a home, finances, and a lot of responsibilities. As a result, the way you act—the character you demonstrate—affects your partner far more profoundly than it did when you were dating.

Many of the things you already do in your day-to-day life can prepare you for your new role as someone's spouse. So, too, the attitudes and behaviors you dis-

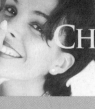

play now are good indicators of how you will act as a spouse.

What follows are common challenges married couples face. As you read about these challenges, think about how you or your potential spouse would handle them. If you've been with your boyfriend or girlfriend long enough, his or her behavior will probably give you a good idea of what to expect after you're married. If you have no idea how your potential spouse would behave, that's a warning sign that you need to learn a lot more about your partner before you get married.

MAINTAINING A HOUSEHOLD

One of the first challenges a newly married couple faces is maintaining a household. In almost any home there are bills to pay, checkbooks to balance, meals to prepare, dishes to wash, clothes to launder, carpets to vacuum, floors to sweep, beds to make, things to fix, and so on.

Maintaining a household provides ample opportunity for conflict. Resentment can flare up quickly when one

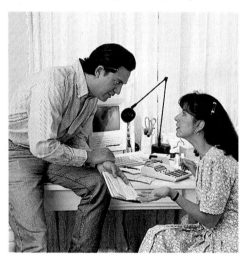

spouse has to do everything because the other refuses to shoulder any responsibility. What would you think, for example, about a wife who doesn't do any work around the house and doesn't work outside the home either? Or a husband who works but won't help his wife at home even when he has the time? You'd probably say that these people are lazy and that their behavior shows a lack of consideration and respect for their mates.

Even when both partners are pulling their weight, clashes can still occur. They may argue over an unpleasant task that neither wants to do—especially if one person is stuck doing it all the time.

Spouses may also differ in their standards of neatness or how often they think things should be done. Let's say, for example, that a newlywed couple named Bill and Maria decide to split the household chores. One of Bill's tasks is cleaning the living room and the bedrooms. He's happy to do his share of work, but he can tolerate more clutter than Maria. As a result, they continually bicker about the way he cleans. Maria is frustrated by all the clutter around the house, while Bill thinks she is being unreasonable.

Good character can play an important role in avoiding quarrels and resentment over maintaining a household. Taking responsibility for your share of the work, showing consideration for your mate, and trying to see things from your mate's point of view can go a long way toward solving and, better yet, preventing problems in this area.

Being a good negotiator also helps. But that doesn't mean getting your way all the time. It means coming to a fair solution that's best for both partners.

Roger Fisher and William Ury, of the

Harvard Negotiation Project, advocate *principled negotiation*. Principled negotiation decides issues "on their merits rather than through a haggling process focused on what each side says it will and won't do. It suggests that you look for mutual gains wherever possible, and that where your interests conflict, you should insist that the result be based on some fair standards independent of the will of either side.... It enables you to be fair while protecting you against those who would take advantage of your fairness."[69]

Over a twenty-year period social psychologist John Gottman has studied the marriages of more than two thousand couples. "A lasting marriage results from a couple's ability to resolve the conflicts that are inevitable in any relationship," he says. "Marriage lives and dies by what you might loosely call its arguments, by how well disagreements and grievances are aired.... The key is how you argue—whether your style escalates tension or leads to a feeling of resolution."[70]

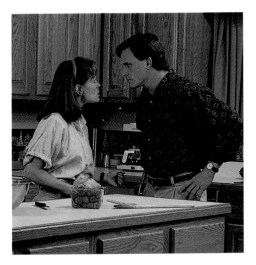

To resolve conflicts, he gives three suggestions:

1. Calm yourself so that you can avoid being negative.
2. Talk and listen without being defensive so that you can have more productive discussions and conflicts.
3. Constantly affirm one another and your relationship even when you have conflict.

Following these steps comes naturally for some people, but most others can learn to do them as well.

"When big problems came up," say Charles and Theresa, married more than sixty-six years, "we talked them over. In loving each other, problems would quickly disappear. The good times we had in the past have outweighed the problems."[71]

John and Joan describe marriage as a partnership: "Like a business, you can't run from problems, so you work them out—laughing at your mistakes and getting on with life." Married forty-six years, this couple has learned to "give in on minor points and never go to bed mad at your spouse."[72]

After forty-five years, John and Carol say they beat the odds because "we both believed in the marriage vows we said to each other." They've also "worked together to overcome any problems." When crises came, this couple says they "endured because we knew the crises wouldn't be long lasting, and we are there for each other, no matter what comes."[73]

MAKING DECISIONS

Another challenge married couples face is making decisions together. One partner's decisions affect the other. If one spouse accepts a job in a distant part of the country, the other will either have to move or live alone most of the year. If one partner makes a big purchase—whether it's a stereo, new furniture, or whatever—the other will have to live with any unpleasant consequences, including financial ones. And that can lead to big fights.

Making a major decision without consulting your spouse sends a strong message of disrespect. When a husband makes a major decision that affects his wife but doesn't consult her, he is saying that he doesn't care how it affects her or that he doesn't think her opinion is worth listening to. Likewise, the wife sends the same message to her husband when she makes a major decision without consulting him.

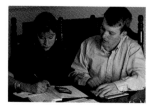

Even when couples make decisions together, there's always the danger that a disagreement will turn into a conflict. Let's say that our newlyweds, Bill and Maria, are discussing a stereo system that Bill saw on sale at a local mall. He wants to buy the system and thinks it's a great bargain. Maria reminds him that they can't afford it and says they should fix the brakes on the car before putting money into a stereo. But Bill can't imagine how anyone could pass up such a great opportunity—and why does Maria always have to be so stingy? Before long the discussion turns to yelling, with Bill storming out of the room and slamming the door behind him.

Peaceful, responsible decision-making takes good character. It requires consideration, looking at things from your spouse's point of view, being a good listener, and being willing to set aside some of your own desires for the good of your spouse.

"We considered ourselves equal partners and were each other's best friend," says Bobbie, a widow after forty-one years of marriage. "If both partners are willing to compromise once in a while, it's way better than losing each other and all you've worked for. We never considered one person better than the other."[74]

"Give and take, and talking things out" helped Gordon and Bea stay married for more than fifty-six years. Having children also made a big difference for them. Perhaps most important, they learned forgiveness: to "forgive each other, even though you might not forget, things that may occur over the years."[75]

As you think about the possibility of marrying someone, look at how you and your potential spouse make decisions. For example, when you go on dates, does one of you try to make all the decisions without consulting the other? Does either of you want things your way all the time and ignore the other's needs or feelings? Does one of you expect the other to go along with everything he or she wants to do? If so, that's something to think about before you say your wedding vows.

Raising Children

Raising children will test your character in almost every way. You may find that you love your children more than you've ever loved anyone in your life. But even that won't keep you from getting stretched to your limits. Children will test your patience. The task of parenting is thus not only rewarding, but often exhausting and frustrating.

During such times most people find it

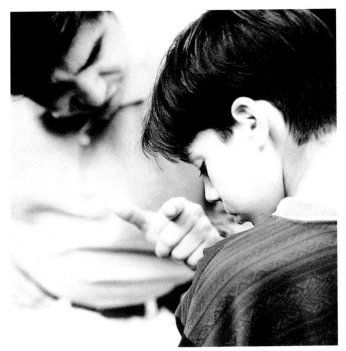

our marriage."[77]

How well do you and your future mate handle fatigue or frustration? Does either of you simply lash out with harsh words—or maybe even physical blows? Are you afraid of your partner when he or she is "stressed out"? Is your partner afraid of you? If so, that's a warning sign you should heed.

SEXUAL FRUSTRATION

One of the advantages of being married is that you and your spouse can enjoy sex whenever you want. That's the theory anyway. In reality it doesn't always work that way.

easy to lose their cool and blow up at each other or at their children. They may say or do things that they later regret or that cause lasting physical or emotional harm. In times of frustration and exhaustion, you'll need patience, self-control, and perseverance.

Many couples blame financial, employment, and child-rearing pressures when they end their marriages. "But the real problem isn't stress," report divorce lawyers in the Family Law Section of the American Bar Association. "It's how a couple handles it—what they expect from each other, how they communicate, how they resolve conflicts."[76]

Married more than fifty years, Glen and Carol say they were serious about their wedding vows and always considered their children. They realized that their children "would be better off with two parents. We didn't want to end

Even in marriage there are many reasons for not having sex. You or your partner may be sick, depressed, angry, too tired, or simply "not in the mood." This can happen when you have young children who take up a lot of your time and energy—and who don't always go to bed when you want them to. Some married couples abstain during those days of the month when the woman is fertile because they are using "natural family planning" to postpone having a child.

Mark and Lisa, the young couple in their mid-twenties mentioned earlier, practiced sexual self-control before marriage and found that they also needed to afterward. They were practicing natural family planning, but there were other considerations as well.

"I think we have a great sex life!" says Lisa. "But anyone who gets married and thinks they're going to have sex every night for the rest of their lives is not living in the real world. And that doesn't just mean couples who have ten kids and are always too worn out by the time they go to bed. People also have jobs, they have school, and they have other commitments.

"Coming into marriage you have to trust that what's important is the quality of the lovemaking," she says, "not the quantity. It really is true that one fantastic night is better than ten when you're exhausted."

Even though Lisa and Mark sometimes come home tired from a busy day, they have both learned to put the other's needs ahead of their own. As Mark pointed out earlier, being one with your partner is the reason for getting married, not just sex.[78]

Handling sexual frustration can be tough. It requires patience and a willingness to back off when your partner says *no*. Physical coercion, of course, is out of the question. But pestering, threats, intimidation, and manipulation are also wrong and can create resentment and ill-will. This is especially true if your spouse simply gives in to your demands.

Before you marry someone, take a good look at how the two of you handle sexual desire. Do you pressure your partner for sex? Does your partner pressure you? Does either one of you come unglued when you don't get your way? If so, that's not likely to change after the wedding. It may even grow worse if one of you thinks you're entitled to have sex whenever you want, regardless of how your partner feels.

On the other hand, practicing sexual self-control right now—before you get married—builds habits that will empower you to respect your partner even when you're frustrated.

SEXUAL TEMPTATION

Like sexual frustration, sexual temptation doesn't end with marriage. Just because it's all right for you to have sex with your partner doesn't mean you won't be tempted by somebody else.

Studies show that the majority of people have successfully resisted such temptation, but many people have not.[79] What's more, the consequences of infidelity are very serious. When you have an affair, you not only break your wedding vow and betray your partner, but you also expose him or her to many of the risks described earlier in this book. Also, marriages in which one or both partners have an affair are far more likely to break up than marriages in which both partners remain faithful.[80]

As with sexual frustration, you can safeguard your future marriage by making a habit of self-control in your current relationships and by thinking about how your actions affect other people. Also, as you put into practice the principles and ideas you learned in the dating chapter, you will become better able to anticipate and avoid situations that put you at risk for infidelity.

FINANCIAL PRESSURES

Financial pressures can put tremendous stress on married couples and are a significant factor in many divorces. Financial pressures have many causes. Sometimes they arise from circumstances beyond the couple's control, such as emergency home or car repairs, medical expenses, disability, or the loss of a job. At other times, however, financial pressures may arise because a couple is careless with money. Either

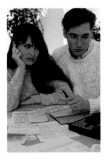

they fail to establish a budget and keep track of their expenses, or they purchase things they don't need and can't afford.

The pressure of major expenses, rising debt, and unpaid bills can be an ongoing source of worry and anxiety, which can spill over into fights. What is worse, if one spouse is trying to keep the finances under control while the other spends money carelessly, the first spouse is bound to resent it.

Imagine that our newlyweds, Bill and Maria, are several thousand dollars in debt—thanks largely to Bill's spending habits. Although Maria buys only the things they absolutely need and passes up a lot of things she would like to get for herself, Bill is continually enticed by new tools, stereo equipment, or computer software. Chances are, it won't be long before she feels cheated by Bill's behavior: Why should *she* be in debt because of his irresponsible spending habits? Why must *she* always be the one to save? Doesn't he care enough about her to help keep their finances under control?

Financial trouble cannot always be avoided by exercising good character, nor is good character always enough to get out of it. But it can certainly help. In fact, responsibility and self-discipline are essential for financial stability. Even in times of financial trouble, exercising these traits will help you avoid needless conflict with your spouse.

How do you and your future spouse handle money? Do you stay within your budget and spend your money wisely? Are you able to pass up things you'd like but can't afford? The answers to these questions could have an important bearing on the happiness of your marriage.

SICKNESS AND INJURY

Just as financial pressures may lead to tough times, health problems or injury may also bring on tough times. Because most people get married when they are young and healthy, they don't usually think about this side of marriage. And that's appropriate because both fun and romance are present in marriage. But deep caring becomes most obvious when

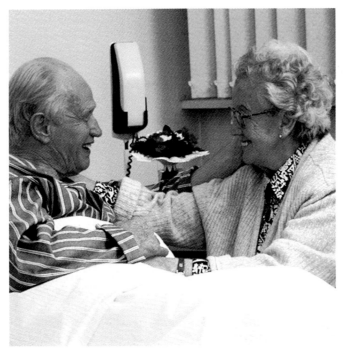

a husband or wife has to pick up the slack for an ailing spouse.

Sometimes you have to look hard to see it, because it often goes on behind the scenes, in bedrooms and hospitals and doctors' offices. But you can see it in the elderly woman who accompanies her husband to the hospital for a battery of frightening heart tests. You can see it in the husband who waits anxiously as his wife undergoes emergency surgery after a terrible car accident. Or in the groggy young wife who drags herself across town in the middle of the night to the only open pharmacy to get a stronger antinausea drug for her husband who is undergoing chemotherapy. Or in the young father who's trying to balance his job, his two young daughters, and his chronically ill wife.

What these and millions of similar scenes reveal are spouses who have set aside their own needs and desires for the good of their partners and their children. Indeed, many of these spouses care for their ailing partners *and* take over the tasks those partners once performed. This kind of caring calls for patience, endurance, and sacrifice.

As you consider marrying someone, it wouldn't hurt to ask yourself if you're the kind of person your future mate could rely on if he or she were seriously ill. You should also ask if your potential spouse is someone you could rely on if *you* became seriously ill.

ARE YOU FIT TO BE TIED?

The attitudes and behaviors you display now are good indicators of how you'll act as a spouse and parent. Listed below are some of the main challenges couples face in marriage and parenthood. One way to prepare yourself for these challenges is to examine your current attitudes and behaviors pertaining to them.

1. MAINTAINING A HOUSEHOLD
   a. Do your parents maintain a household? Whether we like it or not, our attitudes and behavior are often modeled after those of our parents. Their successes and failures are things to watch for in our own relationships.
   b. Have you always expected your mother or father to clean up after you? Do you still expect them to do that today?
   c. Would you be willing to do some of the unpleasant jobs in maintaining a household, including cleaning the bathrooms and refrigerators, mopping the floors, or doing the laundry? Have you ever done any of these jobs?
   d. Do you think any jobs are beneath you or are not your responsibility? For instance, do you think that women should do the cooking and cleaning while men do the repairs and yard work? Are you the kind of person who says, "Hey, that's not my responsibility"?

2. MAKING DECISIONS

a. Arguments and disagreements are part of marriage. How do your parents handle disagreements? How does the way they handle disagreements make you feel? Do you think your parents handle most difficulties successfully? If not, what would you do differently?

b. When you go on dates, do you make most of the decisions without consulting your partner?

c. Do you usually get your way? How do you react when you don't?

3. RAISING CHILDREN

a. With children, love is spelled t-i-m-e. Would you be willing to give up much of your free time to spend it with your children?

b. Parents have to be service-oriented. They have to anticipate their children's needs and think of ways to help them. In what ways do you anticipate the needs of your family members and help them? How do you anticipate the needs of your friends?

c. Meeting your children's needs will frequently require you to set aside your own desires. In what situations have you set aside your desires to meet the needs of others? How did you behave in those situations?

d. In helping children grow, parents have to be patient and forgiving when children make mistakes or fail to meet the parents' expectations. How do you respond when others don't meet your expectations?

e. Parents need humility since children often do things that embarrass their parents in public. How would you respond in such a situation? Do you have any younger brothers or sisters? How do you react when they do things that embarrass you?

f. Parents can make mistakes too. If you made a mistake in front of your child, would you be willing to apologize? Would you be willing to ask your child for forgiveness?

g. Children learn by example. A parent's effectiveness is not merely a matter of words, but deeds. Do you ever find yourself saying one thing but doing another? For instance, do you say you're against drunk drivers, but sometimes drive home drunk? Do you despise liars, but lie when it's convenient? Do you scorn intolerant people, but snub others who don't live up to your expectations?

h. Parenthood demands determination. Determination as a parent means using your energy and willpower to be a good parent even when your efforts seem to be getting nowhere. Do you give up when things get tough, or can you face challenges? Do you settle for things the way they are, such as poor grades, poor relationships, or being out of shape, instead of trying to change your lifestyle and behavior?

   i. Fatigue and frustration are part of parenthood. How do you handle fatigue and frustration?

4. SEXUAL FRUSTRATION AND TEMPTATION

   a. Sexual self-control is a crucial element of any healthy, stable marriage. How good are you, right now, at saying *no* to sexual temptation?

   b. Do you pressure your partner for sex? Does your partner pressure you?

   c. Do you lie and say things you don't really mean so that someone will have sex with you?

   d. Have you told your partner that unless the two of you have sex, you'll never really consider him or her as a potential marriage partner?

   e. Would you abandon your partner for a better-looking, or sexually more available, partner?

5. FINANCIAL PRESSURES

   a. In most marriages the spouses share their resources, including their financial resources. One spouse usually takes care of managing the financial assets. Do you know how to manage your money? Can you draw up a budget and stick to it?

   b. What kind of spending habits do you have? Are you a spender or a saver? Can you pass up things you'd like to have but can't afford?

   c. Are you always short of cash? Do you frequently borrow from others? If you borrow from your friends or parents, how long does it take you to pay them back? Do you have a reputation for not paying people back at all?

6. SICKNESS AND INJURY

   a. What would you do if your fiancé got in a car accident and lost a leg? Would you remain with him?

   b. Could you rely on your partner if you were seriously ill or injured?

   c. What would you do if you found out that your partner was infertile?

   d. If you lost your looks, would your dating relationship continue?

   e. Would you marry your fiancée if she became blind before the wedding?

   f. The word *compatibility* means more than getting along with someone or having things in common. Compatibility comes from the same word as compassion, which means to suffer and endure tough times together. When you face tough times with a friend, a family member, or a dating partner, do you hang in there together? How well do you endure tough times?

Divorce is so widespread in America that many people doubt their own chances for having a successful marriage. Even so, you can do many things that will greatly improve your chances for a healthy, lifelong marriage.

From his studies of marriage and family life, David Popenoe recommends three steps that people should take when considering marriage:[81]

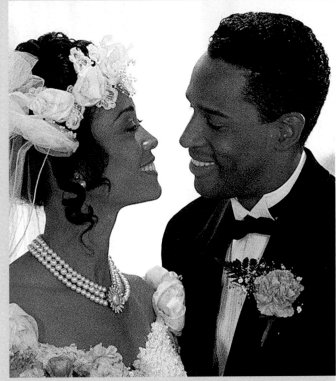

- **Marry at an older age.** "Age at marriage has proven to be one of the single most important predictors of eventual divorce, with the highest divorce rates found among those who marry in their teenage years," according to Dr. Popenoe. In fact, the chances for divorce are considerably less for people who marry in their early twenties than for people who marry in their teens. The chances for divorce are even lower for people who marry in their mid-to-late twenties. Maturity, knowing better what you want in a mate and being more settled in a job or career are among the reasons why later marriages last longer.

- **Choose a mate with your head as much as with your heart.** "Love is not enough," cautions Dr. Popenoe. "Ideally, one is marrying not only a sexual partner but a best friend." Some factors to consider when choosing a mate include how well you get along with each other and the values, opinions, and beliefs you share.

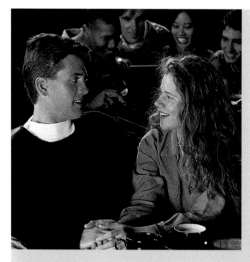

- **Know your partner well for a long time before marrying.** This will help ensure compatibility. Knowing a person for a short time makes it harder for you to sort out incompatible partners. You'll also be less likely to encounter differences that could develop into major problems.

What makes a marriage successful? Here are seven qualities that are usually found in good marriages:[82]

- Ability to change and tolerate change; flexibility.
- Ability to live with the unchangeable; knowing when to seek change and when to accept things the way they are.
- Assumption of permanence; commitment; determination that "this marriage will last."
- Trust, which is the basis of real love and intimacy.
- Balance of responsibilities and power; no master-slave relationship.
- Enjoyment of each other; especially sharing a sense of humor.
- A shared history that is cherished.

WHY SAVING SEX MATTERS

Good character is an important ingredient of successful marriages. Moreover, the way you behave before the wedding vows affects your chances for a successful marriage. Let's take a closer look at how this works in the area of sexuality.

In what was perhaps the most comprehensive survey of sexual behavior in America, researchers at the University of Chicago found that the first marriages of virgins are significantly more stable than the marriages of nonvirgins.[83]

A variety of possible explanations can be given for this finding, but according to these researchers, "those who value virginity and think nonmarital sex inap-propriate also value the commitment to marriage and are disinclined, relatively, to divorce.... [T]hose who are virgins at marriage are those who go to greater lengths to avoid divorce."[84]

In addition, people who have sex before marriage tend to enter into a partnership (either marriage or a live-in relationship) earlier than those who do not, and they are more likely to separate or divorce.[85]

The benefits of saving sex for marriage are by now apparent. Those who wait until marriage don't have to cope with the physical or emotional risks of unwed sex. No rude surprises await in the form of STDs and their aftereffects. Couples who abstain from premarital sex will not be pushed into an early or unwise marriage by an unintended pregnancy—or by guilt over their sexual behavior.

Finally, couples who do not have sex before marriage will have an easier time discerning whether their relationship is based on love or infatuation (see the sidebar "Distinguishing Between Infatuation and Love" in chapter 7). Infatuation can feel very much like love, but it is a poor basis for any lasting relationship. Having sex can inflame your emotions and make it harder to be honest about your relationship.

Establish a good dating relationship without sex. That will free you and your partner to strengthen your trust, love, communication, and friendship. As a result, you'll be able to discern whether you really are meant to spend your lives together. Then when you do get married, sex will become a beautiful bond that ties you together even more tightly.

CONCLUSION

Throughout this book we've seen good reasons why saving sex until marriage will benefit you now and in the future. Even so, you may not fully understand why until you are married.

Lisa didn't. "Before Mark and I got married, our sexuality weighed heavily on me, as I think it does on other young couples. We loved each other so much. But once I was married, it was clear to me why we waited," she says.

Lisa tells her single friends, "You will understand the incredible power that sex has to be a unifying force in your lives— when you're sharing the same checking account, when you're in the same house,

when you have to learn to live with this other person in a million ways. Sex becomes a real celebration of that unity. Before marriage, sex doesn't have that powerful symbolic quality to it."

She also encourages her single friends to wait: "If you do love this person and you are going to get married, sex is going to be better than you ever dreamed of if you wait." Your first contact will then be in the context where sex can be as good as it was meant to be.[86]

Do you remember Norm Cadarette in chapter 1? By sacrificing sexual intimacy with his wife, he showed that love is more than a feeling or pleasure—it's a daily decision. Sometimes love has more to do with suffering than happiness. True love is formed through our willingness to endure tough times together.

Do you remember Armstrong Williams and Melissa Whitaker? They learned that love means respecting yourself and others so much that you do what is right.

You show love by working through the daily strains and stresses in your relationships with family and friends. Showing love includes sticking to your promises, controlling your feelings, and respecting others, treating them the way you want to be treated. As a result, when you date seriously and consider marriage, you will be more likely to control your sexual desires and want what is best for your partner.

Love is important. As Mother Teresa said, "We are created to love, and to be loved."

Love seeks the best for yourself and others. True love, including the sexual dimension of love, becomes yours— a thing of joy and beauty if founded on character.

WHAT IS TRUE LOVE?

A relationship founded on true love is not in danger of falling apart like a relationship founded merely on an emotional bond. Relationships founded on true love are long-lasting. Couples who truly love each other postpone sexual activity until marriage because they know that this is best for them individually and for their relationship. As we've seen, relationships survive longer if sexual activity is postponed until marriage.

What are the foundations for a "true love" relationship? The Greek language has four words for love that help answer this question:

1. **Philia—friendship**: *Philia* (*phi-LEE-uh*) is the love between friends. Good friends like and trust each other. Friendship gives a relationship stability. It helps prevent emotional peaks and valleys. A genuine friend will not try to maneuver you into doing something you don't want to do. True friends won't pressure you to do anything unhealthy or inappropriate (like cheat, lie, or steal). Couples need to be friends before entering a serious relationship. "True love" waits for physical intimacy. Friendship enables a relationship to continue, whether or not the couple marries.

2. **Agape—love**: *Agape* (*ah-GAH-peh*) enables a person to respect and care for others simply because they are human beings, regardless of their imperfections. People with *agape* also recognize their own imperfections. Compatibility, respect, commitment, and unconditional acceptance are all part of *agape*. It is the most important foundation of a true love relationship. Two people in a true love relationship look up to each other and build each other up. *Agape* helps people be their best. It does not try to pull people down or lower their standards. It makes people feel good about themselves. *Agape* meets the needs of others without expecting something in return.

3. **Storge—physical and family affection**: *Storge* (*STOR-geh*) is the love between family members. Young people may not always *feel* love toward a brother or sister. *Storge* enables them to continue to love family members despite passing emotions.

4. **Eros—physical desire**: *Eros*, or erotic love, is physical and sensual love. After a couples marries, sexual activity is added to their relationship similar to the way a roof is added to a house. Just as the roof of a house must be supported by strong walls and a solid foundation, sexual activity requires the strong foundation of marriage (especially one based on shared values and common interests). The marital relationship includes more than physical intimacy. At the same time, sex within marriage strengthens the bond built on friendship, commitment, respect, compatibility, and unconditional acceptance.

A marriage relationship needs all four kinds of love: *philia*, *agape*, *storge*, and *eros*. Not one of the four loves is enough by itself to sustain a happy marriage. When a relationship is based upon true love, it will be able to withstand many problems and crises.

A marriage based on true love also provides the solid foundation needed for parenthood. Successful parenting is easier within a strong, stable, and happy marriage. This has implications for society. The stability of a society is measured by the stability of its families. Strong families and good parents are necessary for a strong and vibrant society.

True love is always a free gift. We give true love hoping that our love will be returned, but without making that a condition of our free gift. True love gives in order to make the person we love happier, healthier, wiser, more mature, more secure, and more content. Its aim is to make the person we love become a better person.

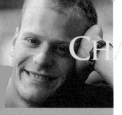

DISCUSSION QUESTIONS

1. Women who save sex for marriage face a lower risk of divorce than women who are sexually active prior to marriage.[87] Why do you think this is the case?

2. What type of spouse will you be? How are you handling your relationships with others now?
   - Are you **generous**? How do you go beyond the minimum in your close relationships?
   - Are you **supportive**? How do you bring out the best in yourself and others?
   - Are you **sensitive**? How much are you aware of the needs and feelings of others?
   - Are you **selfless**? How much do you care about others? Describe one situation where you place others first and yourself second.

3. How are you handling your sexual drives and desires now, before marriage? How will you handle these drives after marriage?

4. You've learned about sexuality from parents, friends, teachers, books, and entertainment, as well as through your own personal life experiences. How have these shaped your views about sexuality?

5. Can you love someone for the rest of your life knowing there will be times when you'll get nothing in return, when your spouse will get mad at you, and when you won't feel like loving?

CHAPTER 1

1. Ginny Cadarette, interview by co-author (D. Cole), 13 September 1996. Basic story from George B. Eager, *Love and Dating* (Valdosta, GA: Mailbox Club Books, 1994), p. 75.

2. Armstrong Williams, "The Power of a Good Name," *Reader's Digest* (Pleasantville, NY: The Reader's Digest Association, March 1996), pp. 63–65.

3. Adapted from Eager, *Love and Dating*, pp. 88–89.

CHAPTER 2

1. *Reader's Digest* (Pleasantville, NY: The Reader's Digest Association, December 1995), pp. 49–55.

2. Thomas Lickona, *Raising Good Children* (NY: Bantam Books, 1983), p. 24.

3. Adapted from George B. Eager, *Love, Dating and Sex* (Valdosta, GA: Mailbox Club Books, 1989), pp. 6–7.

4. Ann Fowler, interview by co-author (M. Duran), October 1996.

5. Neal Shusterman, *Kid Heroes* (NY: Tom Doherty Associates Inc., 1991), pp. 38–39.

6. "Jackie Joyner-Kersee Jumps for Bronze in Her Final Olympic Appearance," article on NBC's Olympic Games Web Site, http://www.olympic.nbc.com/daybyday/802track03.html.

7. Ibid.

8. William Bennett, "The Teacher, the Curriculum, and Values Education Development," in Mary Louise McBee, *New Directions for Higher Education: Rethinking College Responsibilities for Values* (San Francisco: Jossey-Bass, 1980), p. 30.

9. Senator Dan Coats in "Points to Ponder," *Reader's Digest* (Pleasantville, NY: The Reader's Digest Association, June 1996), p. 252.

10. Shusterman, *Kid Heroes*, pp. 43–46.

11. Ibid., pp. 8–11.

12. Margot Stern Strom, "Facing History and Ourselves: Holocaust and Human Behavior," in Ralph Mosher, ed., *Moral Education: A First Generation of Research and Development* (NY: Praeger Publishers, 1980), p. 223.

13. Robert Coles, *The Moral Life of Children* (Boston: Houghton Mifflin Company, 1986), pp. 141–42.

14. Ibid., p. 142.

15. Ibid., p. 143.

16. Ibid.

17. Ibid., p. 144.

18. Ibid., p. 145.

19. Ibid., p. 146.

20. Ibid., pp. 146–47.

21. Ibid., p. 147.

22. Ibid.

23. Ibid., p. 149.

24. Ibid., p. 148.

25. Ibid., p. 150.

26. Ibid., p. 151.

27. Ibid.

28. Ibid., pp. 152–53.

29. Ibid., p. 153.

30. Ibid.

31. Ibid.

32. Ibid., p. 154.

33. George Eager, *Understanding Your Sex Drive* (Valdosta, GA: Mailbox Club Books, 1994), p. 45.

34. Daniel Yankelovich, *New Rules: Searching for Self-Fulfillment in a World Turned Upside Down* (NY: Random House, 1981), p. xviii.

35. William Bennett, *The Index of Leading Cultural Indicators* (NY: Touchstone, 1994), pp. 18–23.

36. United States Department of Justice, Office of the Attorney General, *Combatting Violent Crime, 1992* (Washington, D.C.: U.S. Government Printing Office, 1993).

37. Department of Justice, Federal Bureau of Investigation, *Crime in the U.S. 1991: Juveniles and Violence 1965-1990* (Washington, D.C.: U.S. Government Printing Office, 1992).

38. Bennett, *The Index of Leading Cultural Indicators*, pp. 46–47.

39. The Alan Guttmacher Institute, *Sex and America's Teenagers* (NY: The Alan Guttmacher Institute, 1994), p. 44.

40. U.S. Bureau of the Census, *Statistical Abstract of the United States*, 112th ed. (Washington, D.C.: U.S. Government Printing Office, 1992), p. 44.

41. *Morbidity and Mortality Weekly Report (MMWR)*, 3 February 1995.

42. Centers for Disease Control, National Center for Health Statistics, "Deaths and Death Rates for the 10 Leading Causes of Death in Specified Age Groups, by Race and Sex," *Monthly Vital Statistics Report*, 42(2S), 1993.

43. *MMWR*, 43(RR-11), 1994, pp. 1–20.

44. Ina V. S. Mullis and Gary W. Philips, *The State of Mathematics Achievement: NAEP's 1990 Assessment of the Nation and the Trial Assessment of the States* (Princeton, NJ: Educational Testing Service, 1991).

45. Archie E. Lapointe, Nancy A. Mead, and Janice M. Askew, *Learning Mathematics* (Princeton, NJ: International Assessment of Educational Progress, Educational Testing Service, 1992).

46. Paul E. Barton and Richard J. Coley, *America's Smallest School: The Family* (Princeton, NJ: Educational Testing Service, 1991), p. 3.

47. Barbara Dafoe Whitehead, "Dan Quayle Was Right," *The Atlantic Monthly*, April 1993, p. 80.

48. Ibid., p. 82.

49. Urie Bronfenbrenner, "Discovering What Families Can Do," in David Blankenhorn, Steven Bayme, and Jean Bethke Elshtain, eds., *Rebuilding the Nest: A New Commitment to the American Family* (Milwaukee, WI: Family Service America, 1990), p. 34.

50. Speech given at the Republican National Convention in San Diego, 13 August 1996.

51. Lickona, *Raising Good Children*, p. 28.

CHAPTER 3

1. Suzanne Chazin, "Let's Get Real About Teen Pregnancy," *Reader's Digest* (Pleasantville, NY: The Reader's Digest Association, September 1996), pp. 49-50.

2. S. L. Barron, "Sexual Activity in Girls Under 16 Years of Age," *British Journal of Obstetrics and Gynecology*, 93, 1986, p. 787.

3. United States Department of Health and Human Services, Public Health Service, Office of Population Affairs, "Your Contraceptive Choices for Now, and for Later" (Bethesda, MD: Family Life Information Exchange, 1989).

4. Submitted by a teacher attending the Chicago, IL, Teacher Training Seminar, December 1989.

5. Data from the 1980s reported in *Facts at a Glance*, Child Trends, Washington, D.C., tel. 202-362-5580.

6. The Alan Guttmacher Institute, *Sex and America's Teenagers*, p. 59.

7. Whitehead, "Dan Quayle Was Right," p. 62.

8. This section on pornography was adapted from Tom and Judy Lickona, with William Boudreau M.D., *Sex, Love and You* (Notre Dame, IN: Ave Maria Press, 1994), pp. 109–10.

9. Dolf Zillman and Jennings Bryant, "Effects of Massive Exposure to Pornography," in N. Malamuth and E. Donnerstein, eds., *Pornography and Sexual Aggression* (NY: Academic Press, 1984).

10. Thomas Lickona, "The Neglected Heart," *American Educator*, Summer 1994, p. 37.

11. Quoted in George B. Eager, *All About Peer Pressure* (Valdosta, GA: Mailbox Club Books, 1994), pp. 49–50.

12. "Honor Student Slain; Girlfriend Charged," *The Oneonta Daily Star*, 21 October 1992.

13. Cited in Lickona, *Sex, Love and You*, p. 71.

14. J. Kikuchi, "Rhode Island Develops Successful Intervention Program for Adolescents," *National Coalition Against Sexual Assault Newsletter* (Fall 1988).

15. Eager, *Love, Dating and Sex*, p. 144.

16. Sally Ward, "Acquaintance Rape and the College Social Scene," *Family Relations*, 40, 1991, pp. 65–71.

17. Shirley P. Glass and Thomas L. Wright, "Sex Differences in Type of Extramarital Involvement and Marital Dissatisfaction," *Sex Roles*, 12(9/10), 1985, p. 1102.

18. Ibid.

CHAPTER 4

1. The Alan Guttmacher Institute, *Sex and America's Teenagers*, p. 38.

2. Ibid.

3. Ibid.

4. Ibid., p. 593.

5. Joseph S. McIlhaney Jr., *Safe Sex* (Grand Rapids, MI: Baker Books, 1991), p. 102.

6. Office of Communications, "Pelvic Inflammatory Disease," in National Institute of Allergy and Infectious Diseases [web site], August 1992, available at http://www.niaid.nih.gov/.

7. Office of Women's Health, "Sexually Transmitted Diseases," in the Centers for Disease Control [web site], September 1996, available at http://www.cdc.gov/; "Pelvic Inflammatory Disease," August 1992.

8. Lars Weström and Per-Anders Mådh, "Pelvic Inflammatory Disease," in King K. Holmes, Per-Anders Mådh, P. Frederick Spraling, and Paul J. Wiesner, eds., *Sexually Transmitted Diseases*, 2nd ed. (NY: McGraw-Hill, 1990), p. 598; Willard Cates Jr., "Teenagers and Sexual Risk-Taking: The Best of Times and the Worst of Times," *Journal of Adolescent Health*, 12(2), March 1991, p. 91.

9. Surgeon General's "Report on Acquired Immune Deficiency Syndrome" (Department of Health and Human Services, October 1986), available at www.healthstat.org/ aidsgen.htm.

10. B. Moscicki, M. A. Shafer, S. G. Millstein, C. E. Irwin Jr., and J. Schachter, "The Use and Limitations of Endocervical Gram Stains and Mucopurulent Cervicitis as Predictors for Chlamydia Trachomatis in Female Adolescents," *American Journal of Obstetrics and Gynecology*, 157(1), July 1987.

11. According to the Centers for Disease Control (CDC), "comprehensive surveillance data for non-gonococcal urethritis, genital herpes simplex virus, human papillomavirus, and trichomoniasis are not available. Ongoing trend data are limited to estimates of trends in physicians' office practices provided by the National Disease and Therapeutic Index." From Division of STD Prevention, *Sexually Transmitted Disease Surveillance, 1995* (Atlanta: Centers for Disease Control and Prevention, September 1996).

12. Office of Communications, "An Introduction to Sexually Transmitted Diseases," in National Institute of Allergy and Infectious Diseases [web site], August 1992, available at http://www.niaid.nih.gov/.

13. Office of Communications, "Chlamydial Infections," in National Institute of Allergy and Infectious Diseases [web site], August 1992, available at http://www.niaid.nih.gov/; "Teen Sex and Pregnancy," in The Alan Guttmacher Institute Gateway [web site], July 1996, available at http://www.agi-usa.org/; *Sexual Health Update*, no. 2 (Austin, TX: Medical Institute of Sexual Health, February 1993); Office of Women's Health, "Sexually Transmitted Diseases," 1996.

14. Also called *Neisseria gonorrhoeae*.

15. Office of Communications, "Gonorrhea," in National Institute of Allergy and Infectious Diseases [web site], August 1992, available at http://www.niaid.nih.gov/.

16. "CDC: Syphilis Cases Plummet," Associated Press, 28 May 1997.

17. National Cancer Institute, "NCI/PDQ Physician Statement: Cervical Cancer" in OncoLink [web site], March 1997, available at http://www.cancer.med.upenn.edu.

18. *National Guidelines for Sexuality and Character Education* (Austin, TX: Medical Institute of Sexual Health, 1996), p. 5.

19. Office of Communications, "Human Papillomavirus and Genital Warts," in National Institute of Allergy and Infectious Diseases [web site], June 1992, available at http://www.niaid.nih.gov/.

20. W. Cates, "Teenagers and Sexual Risk-Taking: The Best of Times and the Worst of Times," *Journal of Adolescent Health*, 12(2), March 1991, p. 88.

21. Joseph S. McIlhaney Jr., *Sexual Health Update*, no. 2 (February 1993).

22. H. M. Bauer, Y. Ting, C. E. Greer, J. C. Chambers, C. J. Tashiro, J. Chimera, A. Reginold, and M. M. Maños, "Genital Human Papillomavirus Infection in Female University Students as Determined by a PCR-Based Method," *Journal of the American Medical Association*, 265, 1991, p. 472–77.

23. Office of Communications, "Human Papillomavirus and Genital Warts," June 1992.

24. Ibid.; F. X. Bosch, M. M. Maños, N. Munoz, M. Sherman, A. M. Jansen, J. Peto, M. H. Schiffman, V. Moreno, R. Kurman, K. V. Shah, and the International Biological Study on Cervical Cancer Study Group, "Prevalence of Human Papilloma Virus in Cervical Cancer: A Worldwide Perspective." *Journal of the National Cancer Institute*, 87(11), 1995, pp. 796–802; E. L. Franco, "Cancer Causes Revisited: Human Papilloma Virus and Cervical Neoplasia," *Journal of the National Cancer Institute*, 87(11), 1995, pp. 779–80.

25. K. Syrjänen, M. Väyrynen, O. Castrén, M. Yliskoski, R. Mäntyjärvi, S. Pyrhönen, and S. Saarikoski, "Sexual Behavior of Women with Human Papilloma Virus (HPV) Lesions of the Uterine Cervix," *British Journal of Venereal Disease*, 60, 1984, pp. 243–48.

26. Most cases of genital herpes involve herpes simplex virus II. Herpes simplex virus I, on the other hand, is usually linked to cold sores and fever blisters, but it can also cause genital infections.

27. J. R. Daling, N. S. Weiss, T. G. Hislop, C. Maden, R. J. Coates, K. J. Sherman, R. L. Ashley, M. Beagrie, J. A. Ryan, and L. Corey, "Sexual Practices, Sexually Transmitted Diseases, and the Incidence of Anal Cancer," *New England Journal of Medicine*, 317, 1987, p. 973.

28. F. K. Lee, R. M. Coleman, L. Pereira, P. D. Bailey, M. Tatsuno, and A. J. Nahmais, "Detection of Herpes Simplex Virus Type 2 Specific Antibody with Glycoprotein G," *Journal of Clinical Microbiology*, 22, 1985, p. 642; R. L. Ashley, J. Militoni, F. Lee, A. Nahmais, and L. Corey, "Comparison of Western Blot and gG-Specific Immunodot Enzyme Essay for Detecting HSV-1 and HSV-2 Antibodies in Human Sera," *Journal of Clinical Microbiology*, 26, 1988, p. 662.

29. Office of Communications, "An Introduction to Sexually Transmitted Diseases," 1992.

30. P. L. Goldman, "Face of AIDS," *Newsweek*, 10 August 1987, p. 22.

31. Cited in Eager, *Love, Dating and Sex*, pp. 94–95, from "AIDS, A Special Report," *Vancouver Sun*, 6 June 1987, p. A-1.

32. J. M. Karon, P. S. Rosenberg, G. McQuillan, M. Khare, M. Gwinn, and L. R. Petersen, "Prevalence of HIV infection in the United States, 1984 to 1992," *Journal of the American Medical Association*, 276(2), 1996, pp. 126–31.

33. Centers for Disease Control and Prevention, *HIV/AIDS Surveillance Report*, 8(2), 1996, pp. 1–40.

34. Ibid.

35. The term *HIV-symptomatic disease* refers to those symptoms that were once known as *ARC*, or *AIDS-related complex*.

36. Rick Weiss, "Evidence of Oral Transfer of AIDS Is Seen," *The Washington Post*, 7 June 1996, pp. A-1, A-16.

37. Ibid.

38. Office of Communications, "Human Papillomavirus and Genital Warts," June 1992.

39. *The Unifier*, May 1996. Southeast Polk Community District school newspaper (Altoona, IA), May 1996.

40. Elise F. Jones and Jacqueline D. Forrest, "Contraceptive Failure Rates Based on the 1988 NSG," *Family Planning Perspectives*, 24(1), January/February 1992, pp. 12–19; Elise F. Jones and Jacqueline D. Forrest, "Contraceptive Failure in the United States: Revised Estimates from the 1982 National Survey of Family Growth," *Family Planning Perspectives*, 21(3), May/June 1989, pp. 103–9.

41. R. Glass, M. Vessey, and P. Wiggins, "Use-Effectiveness of the Condom in a Selected Family Planning Clinic Population in the United Kingdom," *Contraception*, 10(6), 1974, pp. 591–98.

42. W. Cates Jr. and K. M. Stone, "Family Planning, Sexually Transmitted Diseases and Contraceptive Choice: A Literature Update—Part I," *Family Planning Perspectives*, 24, 1992, pp. 75–84; "Family Planning, Sexually Transmitted Diseases and Contraceptive Choice: A Literature Update—Part II," *Family Planning Perspectives*, 24, 1992, pp. 122–28.

43. Susan C. Weller, "A Meta-Analysis of Condom Effectiveness in Reducing Sexually Transmitted HIV," *Social Science & Medicine*, 36, June 1993, pp. 1635–44; A. Saracco, M. Musicco, A. Nicolosi, G. Angarano, C. Arici, G. Gavazzeni, P. Costigliola, S. Gafa, C. Gervasoni, R. Luzzati, et al., "Man-to-Woman Sexual Transmission of HIV: Longitudinal Study of 343 Steady Partners of

Infected Men," *Journal of Acquired Immune Deficiency Syndromes*, 6, 1993, pp. 497–502; M. D. Guimaraes, A. Munoz, C. Boschi-Pinto, and E. A. Castilho, "HIV Infection Among Female Partners of Seropositive Men in Brazil," *American Journal of Epidemiology*, 142, 1996, pp. 538–47; I. de Vincenzi, "A Longitudinal Study of Human Immunodeficiency Virus Transmission by Heterosexual Partners," *New England Journal of Medicine*, 331, 1994, pp. 341–46. The study by de Vincenzi showed no transmission of HIV among partners who used condoms consistently, but this appears to be the exception.

44. Cates and Stone, *Family Planning*.

45. Joseph S. McIlhaney Jr., *Sexuality and Sexually Transmitted Diseases* (Grand Rapids, MI: Baker Books, 1990), p. 35.

46. Surgeon General's "Report on Acquired Immune Deficiency Syndrome," October 1986.

47. Personal interview by co-author (M. Duran) with Dr. Elizabeth Hertz, George Washington University Medical Center, Washington, D.C., 23 August 1991.

48. *Division of STD/HIV Prevention, Annual Report*, Department of Health and Human Services, 1990, p. 5.

49. M. Piazza, A. Chiranni, M. Picciotto, V. Guadagnino, R. Orlando, and P. T. Cataldo, "Passionate Kissing and Microlesions of the Oral Mucosa," *Journal of the American Medical Association*, 261, 13 January 1989, pp. 244–45.

CHAPTER 5

1. Chazin, "Let's Get Real About Teen Pregnancy," pp. 52–54.

2. Whitehead, "Dan Quayle Was Right," p. 62.

3. William A. Galston, "Beyond the Murphy Brown Debate," paper presented at the Institute for American Values Family Policy Symposium, NY, 10 December 1993.

4. William Raspberry, "Let's Get Real about Unwed Teenage Moms," *Orlando Sentinel*, 6 September 1996, p. A15.

5. Ibid.

6. David Popenoe, "The Controversial Truth: Two-Parent Families Are Better," *The New York Times*, 26 December 1992, p. D21.

7. National Committee for Adoption, *Adoption Factbook: United States Data, Issues, Regulations and Resources* (Washington, D.C.: National Committee for Adoption, 1989), cover.

8. Ibid., p. 127.

9. Edmund Mech, "Orientations of Pregnancy Counselors Toward Adoption," study conducted for the Office of Adolescent Pregnancy Prevention, 1989. Cited in *Adoption Factbook*, p. 143.

10. *Adoption Factbook*, p. 148; Project Share, *The Adoption Option: A Guidebook for Pregnancy Counselors* (U.S. Department of Health and Human Services, Office of Population Affairs, and Office of the Assistant Secretary for Planning and Evaluation), 1986, p. 16; C. A. Bachrach, "Adoption Plans, Adopted Children and Adoptive Mothers," *Journal of Marriage and the Family*, 48, May 1986, pp. 243–53.

11. *The Adoption Option*, p. 16; Bachrach, *Journal of Marriage and the Family*.

12. *Adoption Factbook*, pp. 157–59; *The Adoption Option*, p. 15.

13. Kathleen Silber and Phylis Speedlin, *Dear Birthmother: Thank You for Our Baby*, foreword by Alberto C. Serrano (San Antonio, TX: Corona Publishing Co., 1982), pp. 113–16.

14. Ibid., pp. 137–38.

15. Ibid., pp. 105–6.

16. Ibid., pp. 66–67.

17. Teen Choice Survey, 6201 Leesburg Pike, Falls Church, VA, 1990.

18. The Alan Guttmacher Institute, "Induced Abortion," *Facts in Brief* (NY: The Alan Guttmacher Institute, January 1997); available at http://www.agi-usa.org.

19. The Alan Guttmacher Institute, *Sex and America's Teenagers*, p. 44.

20. Ibid.

21. E. Joanne Angelo, "The Negative Impact of Abortion on Women and Families," in Michael T. Mannion, ed., *Post-Abortion Aftermath* (Kansas City, MO: Sheed & Ward, 1994), p. 51.

22. Ibid., p. 52.

23. Ibid., p. 55.

24. Ibid., p. 52.

25. Ibid., p. 44.

26. Ibid.

27. Ibid.

28. Joyce Price, "Statistics May Be Misleading on Deaths Caused by Abortion," *The Washington Times*, 4 June 1994, p. A5.

29. Report of Investigation by Medical Examiner, Case No. 93-1948; North Carolina Medical Examiner's Certificate of Death, Vital Records No. 044550, issued 12 October 1993.

30. Alabama Certificate of Death, File No. 85-10613.

CHAPTER 6

1. Chazin, "Let's Get Real About Teen Pregnancy," pp. 51–52.

2. Whitehead, "Dan Quayle Was Right," p. 62.

3. Thomas Lickona, "The Neglected Heart," p. 35, from "Some Teens Taking Vows of Virginity," *Washington Post*, 21 November 1993.

4. Ibid.

5. Eager, *Love, Dating and Sex*, p. 73.

6. Dick Purnell, *Becoming a Friend and Lover* (San Bernardino, CA: Here's Life Publishers, 1986), p. 54.

7. Adapted from Eager, *Love, Dating and Sex*, pp. 6–7.

8. Lickona, "The Neglected Heart," p. 37.

9. Ray E. Short, *Sex, Love or Infatuation* (Minneapolis, MN: Augsburg Publishing House, 1978), p. 98.

10. Lickona, "The Neglected Heart," p. 36.

11. Ibid.

12. "Casual Sex on Campus Declines," *USA Today*, 10 January 1985.

13. Lickona, "The Neglected Heart," p. 36.

14. Ibid., p. 37.

15. Personal interview by co-author (M. Duran), Marymount College, Fredericksburg, VA, 1994.

16. Lickona, "The Neglected Heart," p. 37.

17. Eager, *Love, Dating and Sex*, p. 179, from Ann Landers, *Ann Landers Talks to Teenagers About Sex* (Englewood Cliffs, NJ: Prentice-Hall, 1963), p. 35.

18. Lickona, "The Neglected Heart," p. 38.

19. Ibid.

20. Ibid., p. 39.

21. Ibid.

22. Ibid., p. 38.

23. Character-Based Education Survey, conducted by co-author (M. Duran) for Family

Life Education, A Choice in Education, Chantilly, VA, February 1995.

24. Kevin Leman, *Smart Kids, Stupid Choices* (Ventura, CA: Regal Books, 1982), p. 95.

25. Dolf Zillman and Jennings Bryant, "Pornography's Impact on Sexual Satisfaction," *Journal of Applied Social Psychology*, 18, 1988, p. 450.

26. A. James Reichley, *Religion in American Public Life* (Washington, D.C.: The Brookings Institution, 1985).

27. George Gallup Jr. and Jim Castelli, *The People's Religion: American Faith in the 90s* (NY: Macmillan Publishing Company, 1989).

28. Lickona, "The Neglected Heart," p. 39.

29. Antonia Abbey, "Sex Differences in Attributions for Friendly Behavior: Do Males Misperceive Females' Friendliness?," *Journal of Personality and Social Psychology*, 42(5), 1982, p. 830.

CHAPTER 7

1. Joe White, *Over the Edge and Back* (Sisters, OR: Questar Publishers, 1992), pp. 30–31.

2. Eager, *Love, Dating and Sex*, pp. 153–54.

3. Elizabeth Thomson and Ugo Colella, "Cohabitation and Marital Stability: Quality or Commitment?," *Journal of Marriage and the Family*, 54, 1992, p. 178.

4. From personal interview with co-author (M. Duran), 24 July 1991.

CHAPTER 8

†Robert T. Michael, John H. Gagnon, Edward O. Laumann, Gina Kolata, *Sex in America, A Definitive Survey* (NY: Little, Brown and Company, 1994), p. 230.

1. Eager, *Understanding Your Sex Drive*, pp. 90–92.

2. Some states allow common law marriages, which involve neither a formal ceremony nor the taking of vows. Despite the absence of a formal ceremony, however, common law marriages are still subject to regulation. In those states that allow it, a common law marriage exists when 1) a couple makes an agreement to be married, 2) the couple lives together as husband and wife, and 3) the couple presents themselves to others as married. Additionally, common law marriages entail the same rights and obligations as other marriages.

3. Some states have gone even further and adopted the Uniform Desertion and Non-Support Act, which requires all husbands to support both wives and any of their children who are under sixteen years old. Failure to do so is a crime in these states.

4. David W. Murray, "Poor Suffering Bastards," *Policy Review*, 68, Spring 1994, p. 13.

5. Edward O. Laumann, John H. Gagnon, Robert T. Michael, and Stuart Michaels, *The Social Organization of Sexuality: Sexual Practices in the United States* (Chicago: The University of Chicago Press, 1994), p. 364.

6. Ibid., p. 365.

7. David Popenoe, *Life Without Father* (NY: Free Press, 1996), p. 217; Laumann et al., *The Social Organization of Sexuality*.

8. Quoted in Richard John Neuhaus, "The Public Square," *First Things*, 43, May 1994, pp. 63–76.

9. Lickona, *Sex, Love and You*, pp. 161–62.

10. David G. Myers, *The Pursuit of Happiness* (NY: William Morrow, 1992), p. 83.

11. Ibid., p. 84.

12. John Guidubaldi and Helen Cleminshaw, "Divorce, Family Health and Child Adjustment," *Family Relations*, 34, 1985, pp. 35–41.

13. Marc L. Berk and Amy K. Taylor, "Women and Divorce: Health Coverage, Utilization and Health Care Expenditures," *American Journal of Public Health*, 74, 1984, pp. 1276–78.

14. Catherine K. Reissman and Naomi Gerstel, "Marital Dissolution and Health: Do Males or Females Have Greater Risk?," *Social Science and Medicine*, 20, 1985, pp. 627–35.

15. Robert H. Coombs, "Marital Status and Personal Well-Being: A Literature Review," *Family Relations*, 40, 1991, pp. 97–102.

16. Popenoe, *Life Without Father*, p. 215.

17. Angus Campbell, *The Sense of Well-Being in America* (NY: McGraw-Hill, 1981), p. 197.

18. Popenoe, *Life Without Father*, p. 216.

19. Maradee A. Davis, John M. Neuhaus, Deborah J. Moritz, and Mark R. Segal, "Living Arrangements and Survival Among Middle-Aged and Older Adults in the NHANES I Epidemiologic Follow-up Study," *American Journal of Public Health*, 82, 1992, pp. 401–6.

20. Myers, *The Pursuit of Happiness*, p. 83.

21. Coombs, "Marital Status," pp. 97–98.

22. Ibid., p. 97.

23. Sanders Korenman and David Neumark, "Does Marriage Really Make Men More Productive?," *Journal of Human Resources*, 26, 1990, pp. 282–307.

24. Catherine E. Ross, "Reconceptualizing Marital Status as a Continuum of Social Attachment," *Journal of Marriage and the Family*, 57(1), 1995, pp. 129–40.

25. Jan E. Stets, "The Link Between Past and Present Intimate Relationships," *Journal of Family Issues*, 14, 1993, pp. 236–60.

26. Kersti Yilo and Murray A. Straus, "Interpersonal Violence Among Married and Cohabiting Couples," *Family Relations*, 30, 1981, pp. 339–47.

27. Stets, "The Link Between Past and Present Intimate Relationships," p. 674.

28. William G. Axinn and Arland Thornton, "The Relationship between Cohabitation and Divorce: Selectivity or Casual Influence?," *Demography*, 29, 1992, pp. 357–74.

29. Neil G. Bennett, Ann Blanc Klimas, and David E. Bloom, "Commitment and the Modern Union: Assessing the Link Between Premarital Cohabitation and Subsequent Marital Stability," *American Sociological Review*, 53, 1988, pp. 127–38.

30. Popenoe, *Life Without Father*, p. 217.

31. See Aaron Hass, *The Gift of Fatherhood: How Men's Lives Are Transformed by Their Children* (NY: Simon and Schuster, 1994); Michael E. Lamb, J. H. Pleck, and J. A. Levine, "The Effects of Paternal Involvement on Fathers and Mothers," in Robert A. Lewis and Marvin B. Sussman, eds., *Men's Changing Roles in the Family* (NY: Haworth, 1986).

32. Ross D. Parke, *Fathers* (Cambridge, MA: Harvard University Press, 1981), p. 11.

33. John Snarey, *How Fathers Care for the Next Generation: A Four-Decade Study*, (Cambridge, MA: Harvard University Press, 1993), pp. 114–18.

34. Campbell, 1981, p. 231.

35. Popenoe, *Life Without Father*, pp. 197–98.

36. Eleanor Baugher and Leatha Lamison-White, "Poverty in the United States: 1995," *Current Population Reports*, Series P60-194 (Washington, D.C.: U.S. Government Printing Office, 1996), p. viii.

37. Ibid., p. vi.

38. Popenoe, *Life Without Father*, p. 139.

39. Murray, "Poor Suffering Bastards," p. 13.

40. Ibid., pp. 9–10.

41. Paul E. Barton and Richard J. Coley, *America's Smallest School: The Family* (Princeton, NJ: Educational Testing Service, 1991), p. 6.

42. Sheila Fitzgerald Krein and Andrea H. Beller, "Educational Attainment of Children From Single-Parent Families: Differences by Exposure, Gender and Race," *Demography*, 25, 1988, p. 228.

43. Travis Hirschi, "Family Structure and Crime," in Bryce J. Christensen, ed., *When Families Fail: The Social Cost* (NY: University Press of America, 1991), p. 56.

44. Ibid.

45. Virginia Department of Health, *Fatherhood and Family Health*, A Survey of Programs Throughout the United States (Virginia Department of Health, Health Policy Group and Division of Child and Adolescent Health, September 1995), p. 6.

46. Ibid.

47. Nicholas Zill, Donna Morrison, and Mary Jo Coiro, "Long-Term Effects of Parental Divorce on Parent-Child Relationships, Adjustment and Achievement in Young Adulthood," *Journal of Family Psychology*, 7, 1993, pp. 1, 91, 100.

48. Virginia Department of Health, *Fatherhood and Family Health*, p. 5.

49. Virginia Department of Health, *Fatherhood and Family Health* p. 4; Deborah A. Dawson, "Family Structure and Children's Health and Well-Being: Data from the National Health Interview Survey on Child Health," *Journal of Marriage and the Family*, 53, 1991, pp. 573–84.

50. Ronald Angel and Jacqueline Lowe Worobey, "Single Motherhood and Children's Health," *Journal of Health and Social Behavior*, 29, 1988, pp. 38, 45.

51. Dawson, 1991, pp. 578–79.

52. Ibid.

53. Ibid.

54. Dawson, "Family Structure."

55. Ibid.

56. Dawson, "Family Structure," pp. 578–79.

57. Judith S. Wallerstein, "The Long-Term Effects of Divorce on Children: A Review," *Journal of the American Academy of Child and Adolescent Psychiatry*, 30, 1991, p. 352.

58. Ibid.

59. Ibid., pp. 352–53, 355.

60. I. Garfinkel and Sarah S. McLanahan, *Single Mothers and Their Children: A New American Dilemma* (Washington, D.C.: The Urban Institute Press, 1986), pp. 30–31.

61. M. Anne Hill and June O'Neill, *Underclass Behaviors in the United States: Measurements and Analysis of Determinants* (NY: City University of New York, Baruch College, 1993), p. 90.

62. James Q. Wilson, "Culture Incentives and the Underclass," in *Values and Public Policy*, Henry J. Aaron, Thomas E. Mann, and Timothy Taylor, eds. (Washington, D.C.: Brookings Institute, 1994), pp. 54–80.

63. Douglas Smith and G. Roger Jarjoura, "Social Structure and Criminal Victimization," *Journal of Research in Crime and Delinquency*, 25, 1988, p. 47.

64. Ibid., pp. 87–88; Edward L. Wells and Joseph H. Rankin, "Families and Delinquency: A Meta-Analysis of the Impact of Broken Homes," *Social Problems*, 38, 1991, p. 87.

65. Virginia Department of Health, *Father-hood and Family Health*, p. 5.

66. Ibid., p. 14.

67. D. Finkelhorn, G. T. Hotaling, and A. J. Sedlack, "Missing, Abducted, Runaway and Thrown Away Children in America," U.S. Department of Justice, Office of Juvenile Justice and Delinquency Prevention, *Executive Summary*, May 1990.

68. Virginia Department of Health, *Father-hood and Family Health*, p. 6.

69. Roger Fisher and William Ury, *Getting to Yes: Negotiating Agreement without Giving In* (NY: Penguin Books, 1981), p. xii.

70. John Gottman, *Why Marriages Succeed or Fail* (NY: Simon and Schuster, 1994), pp. 28, 173.

71. Personal interview by co-author (D. Cole), Apopka, FL, September 1996.

72. Ibid.

73. Ibid.

74. Ibid.

75. Ibid.

76. Popenoe, *Life Without Father*, pp. 208–9. For further information, contact the American Bar Association's Family Law Section at 750 Lake Shore Drive, Chicago, IL 60611.

77. Personal interview by co-author (D. Cole), Apopka, FL, September 1996.

78. Lickona, p. 174.

79. Laumann et al., *The Social Organization of Sexuality*, p. 214.

80. Ibid., p. 215.

81. Popenoe, *Life Without Father*, pp. 201–2.

82. Ibid., p. 206.

83. Laumann et al., *The Social Organization of Sexuality*, p. 503.

84. Ibid., p. 505.

85. Ibid.

86. Lickona, p. 174.

87. Joan R. Kahn and Kathryn A. London, "Premarital Sex and the Risk of Divorce," *Journal of Marriage and the Family*, 53, 1991, pp. 845–55.

Maureen Gallagher Duran—Co-author. B.S. in Political Science, Radford University, 1983; Teaching Certificate, George Mason University, 1986; M.A. in Education and Counseling, George Mason University, 1987. Director for 10 years of Education of Teen Choice, a project funded in part by the Office of Adolescent Pregnancy Programs, U.S. Department of Health and Human Services. Author of nationally recognized secondary high school, family-life/sexuality curriculum, *Reasonable Reasons to Wait (RRTW)*. Author of peer education and mentoring program, Peers Assisted Learning (PAL). Author of middle school curriculum, *Character Counts: Making the Right Moves*. Author of Teacher's Guide to video, *Sex, Lies and the Truth*. Author of *Character Building Skits for the Elementary*. Recognized speaker in the field of character-based sexuality education.

Deborah D. Cole–Co-author. B.A. in Sociology, University of Maryland, 1971; M.A. in Communications, Regent University, 1980; post-graduate studies in mass communication, Regent University, 1980; post-graduate studies in education, Old Dominion University, 1982; studies in literature, Rollins College, 1994-1997. Editor, *Handbook for Helping Others*, by Kenneth Stafford, Chosen Books, Zondervan Corporation, 1986. Managing Editor, Strang Communications, 1988-1995. Writer, instructor at writers' conferences.

William A. Dembski—Academic Editor. Ph.D., Mathematics, University of Chicago; Ph.D., Philosophy, University of Illinois at Chicago; M.Div., Princeton Theological Seminary; writer, lecturer, author of *The Design Inference* (Cambridge University Press, 1998) and editor of *Mere Creation: Science, Faith, and Intelligent Design* (InverVarsity Press, 1998). Post-doctoral work at MIT, University of Chicago, Northwestern, Princeton, Cambridge, and Notre Dame. National Science Foundation doctoral and post-doctoral fellow. Publications range from mathematics (*Journal of Theoretical Probability*) to philosophy (*Nous*) to theology (*Scottish Journal of Theology*). Fellow of the Discovery Institute's Center for the Renewal of Science and Culture.

Joe S. McIlhaney, Jr., M.D.—Foreword. Board certified obstetrician/gynecologist. Active on the medical staff of St. David's Community Hospital, Austin, TX. Special work on reproductive technologies, contraceptive techniques, sexuality education, sexually transmitted diseases and social behavior education. Instrumental, with three other physicians, in bringing in-vitro fertilization and embryo transfer to Austin. In 1992, established the Medical Institute for Sexual Health, a non-profit research organization. Left private practice in 1995 to devote full attention to working with the Institute. Speaker and writer about the twin epidemics of STDs and nonmarital pregnancy. Author of six books including *1250 Health-Care Questions Women Ask* and his latest publication, *Sex: What You Don't Know Can Kill You*.

Front Cover: Mel Di Giacomo/ The Image Bank (TIB)

Chapter Openings: David De Lossy/ TIB, Barros & Barros/TIB, David M. Grossman/Phototake NYC, Greg Weiner/Tony Stone Images, Ed Malitsky/Tony Stone Images, Barros & Barros/TIB, Ron Krisel/Tony Stone Images, David Vance/TIB

Page: Ross Whitaker/TIB, David De Lossy/TIB, Simon Wilkinson/TIB, David Young-Woltt/Tony Stone Images, Vicky Kasala/TIB, Stephen Whalen/Uniphoto, Alan Becker/TIB, David De Lossy/TIB, Flip Chalfant/TIB, Butch Martin/TIB, David De Lossy/TIB, Butch Martin/TIB, Maria Taglienti/TIB, Mel Di Giacomo/TIB, Bob Daemmrich/ Uniphoto, Bob Daemmrich/Uniphoto, Benn Mitchell/TIB, Vicky Kasala/TIB, David De Lossy/TIB, David De Lossy/ TIB, David De Lossy/TIB, Bob Daemmrich/Uniphoto, David De Lossy/TIB, Yuri Cojc/TIB, Carol Kohen/TIB, David De Lossy/TIB, S. Dunwell/TIB, Bob Daemmrich/ Uniphoto, Steve Allen/TIB, Barros & Barros/TIB, Llewellyn/Uniphoto, Yellow Dog Prods/TIB, C. Gordon/TIB, Michael Keller/Uniphoto, Jeff Hunter/ TIB, Jeff Dunas/TIB, David De Lossy/ TIB, Vicky Kasala/TIB, Barros & Barros/TIB, Jim Olive/Uniphoto, Mark's Product/TIB,Chris M. Rogers/ TIB, David De Lossy/TIB, Regine M./TIB, Flip Chalfant/TIB, David De Lossy/TIB, Henley & Savage/Uniphoto, David De Lossy/TIB, Llewellyn/ Uniphoto, Butch Martin/TIB, Jeffry W. Myers/Uniphoto, Llewellyn/Uniphoto, Garry Gay/TIB, Daniel Grogan/ Uniphoto, John Henley/Uniphoto, Llewellyn/Uniphoto, Jon Fenigersh/ Uniphoto, Barros & Barros/TIB, Yellow Dog Prods/TIB, Llewellyn/Uniphoto, A. Broccaccio/TIB, Barros & Barros/TIB, David Hamilton/TIB, Bachmann/ Uniphoto, J.B. Smith/Uniphoto, Busi/Comm/Uniphoto, Michael Keller/Uniphoto, Llewellyn/Uniphoto, Penny Tweedie/Tony Stone Images, David Young Wolff/ Tony Stone Images, Christopher Bisssell/Tony Stone Images, Mitch York/Tony Stone Images, Eric Larrayadieu/Tony Stone Images, Erica Lansner/Tony Stone Images, Rosanne Olson/Tony Stone Images, Penny Tweedie/Tony Stone Images, I. Burgum/P Boorman/Tony Stone Images, David Young Wolff/ Tony Stone Images, Zigy Kaluzny/Tony Stone Images, Bob Thoms/Tony Stone Images, Jim Craigmyle/Masterfile, Zigy Kaluzny/Tony Stone Images, David Tejada/Tony Stone Images, H.G. Ross/Masterfile, Color Day/TIB, Jay Freis/TIB, Marc Grinberg/TIB, Kevin Horan/Tony Stone Images, Bob Daemmrich/Uniphoto, Steve Wanke/ Uniphoto, Frank Fitman/Uniphoto, David Stover/Uniphoto, Bob Daemmrich/Uniphoto, Michael Keller/Uniphoto